VB6

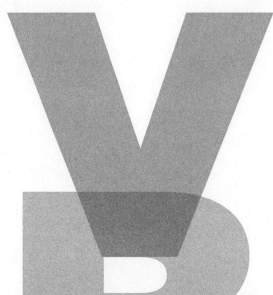

THE FLEXIBLE DIET YOU CAN REALLY STICK TO,
WITH MORE THAN 60 EASY, DELICIOUS RECIPES

EAT VEGAN BEFORE 6:00

TO LOSE WEIGHT AND
RESTORE YOUR HEALTH...
FOR GOOD

MARK BITTMAN

FOREWORD BY
DEAN ORNISH, M.D.

CLARKSON POTTER/PUBLISHERS
NEW YORK

OTHER BOOKS BY MARK BITTMAN

Fish: The Complete Guide to Buying and Cooking

Leafy Greens

How to Cook Everything

How to Cook Everything Vegetarian

How to Cook Everything: The Basics

How to Cook Everything: Bittman Takes on America's Chefs

The Best Recipes in the World

Food Matters

The Food Matters Cookbook

The Minimalist Cooks Dinner

The Minimalist Cooks at Home

The Minimalist Entertains

Mark Bittman's Quick and Easy Recipes from the New York Times

The Mini Minimalist

Published in the United States by Clarkson Potter/Publishers, an imprint of the
Crown Publishing Group, a division of Random House, Inc., New York.
www.crownpublishing.com   www.clarksonpotter.com

CLARKSON POTTER is a trademark and POTTER with colophon is a
registered trademark of Random House, Inc.

"VB6" and "VEGAN BEFORE SIX" are trademarks of Double B Publishing, Inc.,
and may not be used without a license agreement from the owner.

Library of Congress Cataloging-in-Publication Data
Bittman, Mark.
VB6: Eat Vegan Before 6:00 p.m. to Lose Weight and Restore Your Health . . . for Good /
Mark Bittman.—First edition.
1. Vegan cooking. 2. Breakfasts. 3. Luncheons. I. Title.
II. Title: Eat vegan before 6:00 p.m.
TX837.B5278   2013
641.5'636—dc23   2012046866

ISBN 978-0-385-34474-6
eISBN 978-0-385-34475-3

Printed in the United States of America

Jacket design by Evan Gaffney Design

3 5 7 9 10 8 6 4 2

First Edition

FOR
SIDNEY M. BAKER

Contents

Foreword

BY DEAN ORNISH

I'm an unabashed admirer of Mark Bittman's work. And when you read this book, chances are you will be, too.

Mark is one of the rare people who thinks clearly, writes courageously, and explains eloquently. In my experience, people who have really mastered a subject can make it simple without being simplistic—not out of ignorance but from a profound and deep understanding.

That's what makes *VB6* such a great book.

There is a convergence of forces that make this the right book, right now. At a time when the limitations of high-tech medicine such as drugs and surgery are becoming clearer and the costs are unsustainable, the power of low-tech approaches such as what we eat are becoming more well-documented than ever.

For the past thirty-six years, my colleagues at the nonprofit Preventive Medicine Research Institute and the University of California, San Francisco, have conducted research proving the power of a whole foods, plant-based diet in combination with stress management techniques, moderate exercise like walking, and love and intimacy. In addition to *preventing* many chronic diseases, these comprehensive lifestyle changes can often stop and even *reverse* the progression of these illnesses, including coronary heart disease, early-stage prostate cancer, and Type 2 diabetes.

We found that changing lifestyle actually changes your genes—turning on genes that keep you healthy, and turning off genes that promote heart disease, prostate cancer, breast cancer, and diabetes—hundreds of genes in just three months. These diet and lifestyle changes can even lengthen your telomeres, the ends of your chromosomes that control aging. As your telomeres get longer, your life gets longer. People often say, "Oh, it's all in my genes; there's not much I can do about it." Knowing that changing lifestyle changes our genes is often very motivating—not to blame, but to empower.

When I began doing this work, I thought that younger people who had less severe disease would do better, but I was wrong. One of the most provocative findings in all of our studies was this: *The more people changed their diet and lifestyle, the better they felt and the more they improved in ways we could measure.* At *any* age.

This is the scientific basis of VB6. It's not all or nothing. You have a spectrum of choices.

I find this message to be extraordinarily empowering—and a crucial tool for people to make sustainable changes in their lifestyle. Since the biological mechanisms that control human health and well-being are so dynamic, when you begin to eat and live healthier, you usually feel so much better, so quickly, that it reframes the reason for change from fear of dying (which is not sustainable) to joy of living (which is).

If you go *on* a diet, you're like to go *off* the diet. Diets are all about what you *can't* have and what you *must* do.

I've learned that even more than feeling healthy, most people want to feel free and in control. If I say, "Always eat this" and "Never eat that," it often makes people want to do exactly the opposite. This goes back to "Don't eat the apple," which didn't turn out very well—and that was God talking.

What matters most is your *overall* way of living and eating. If you indulge yourself one day, it doesn't mean you cheated or failed; just eat healthier the next. This way, you can't fail.

Mark Bittman understands this. The more you change your diet and lifestyle, the better you feel and the healthier you become.

If you eat vegan before dinner and indulge yourself afterward, you're likely to notice great improvements in your health and well-being without feeling deprived. As you start to feel better and notice how much healthier you are, you're likely to find yourself in a virtuous cycle in which you may want to do even more.

Of course, you could just as easily say you want to be vegan *after* 6:00 p.m. as before and you're also likely to get good results. Or vegan on alternating days. Or just have meatless Mondays.

You get the idea.

You decide how much you want to change your diet, and how quickly. If that degree of change is enough to accomplish your goals, then that's all you need to do. If not, you can do more.

Radically simple.

In addition to personal health benefits, the food choices we make each day affect other important areas as well. What's personally sustainable is globally sustainable. What's good for you is good for our planet.

As Mark Bittman describes here, eating a vegan diet, even part-time, can have an important impact on issues like global warming, health care costs, and energy conservation. This makes our dietary choices even more meaningful and, thus, more sustainable.

For example, many people are surprised to learn that animal agribusiness—eating meat—generates more greenhouse gases than all forms of transportation *combined.*

More than half of U.S. grain and nearly 40 percent of world grain is being fed to livestock rather than being consumed directly by humans. More than 8 billion livestock are maintained in the U.S., which eat about seven times as much grain as consumed by the entire U.S. population.

At a time when 20 percent of people in the United States go to bed hungry each night and almost 50 percent of the world's population is malnourished, choosing to eat more plant-based foods and less red meat is better for all of us—ourselves, our loved ones, and our planet.

More than 75 percent of the $2.8 trillion in annual U.S. health-care costs are from chronic diseases which often can be prevented and even reversed by eating a plant-based diet at a fraction of the costs.

And the only side effects are good ones.

Dean Ornish, M.D.
Founder and President, Preventive Medicine Research Institute
Clinical Professor of Medicine, University of California, San Francisco
author of *The Spectrum*
www.ornish.com

Introduction

Six years ago, the man I most trusted with my health said to me, "You should probably become a vegan."

Not exactly the words I'd wanted to hear, and certainly not what I was expecting. But I'd asked Sid Baker, my doctor of thirty years, what he recommended, given that he'd just told me that at age 57, I had developed the pre-diabetic, pre-heart-disease symptoms typical of a middle-aged man who'd spent his life eating without discipline.

He'd laid out the depressing facts for me: "Your blood numbers have always been fine but now they're not. You weigh 40 pounds more than you should. You're complaining of sleep apnea. You're talking about knee surgery, which is a direct result of your being overweight. Your cholesterol, which has always been normal up until now, isn't. Same with your blood sugar; it's moved into the danger zone."

A more conventional doc would've simply put me on a drug like Lipitor, and maybe a low-fat diet. But Lipitor, one of the statin drugs that lowers cholesterol, is a permanent drug: Once you start taking it, you don't stop. I didn't like the idea of that. Furthermore, its effectiveness in healthy people has never been established, and it's also been implicated in memory loss and other cognitive complications; I didn't like the idea of any of that, either. And at this point, low-fat and low-carbohydrate diets have essentially been discredited: They might help you lose weight, but they're not effective for maintaining that loss in the long term, and they may even wreak havoc on your system.

But becoming a vegan? A person who eats no animal products at all? Calling that a radical change to my lifestyle was more than a bit of an understatement. Yet it was clear that something had to be done. I asked Sid, "Is a compromise possible? Any other ideas?"

"You're a smart guy," he said. "Figure something out."

I thought about this for a few days, and I recognized that what he was saying made sense. There are no silver bullets, and over the years it's become increasingly clear—much as none of us wants to hear it—that the most sensible diet for human health and longevity is one that's lower in animal products and junk food and higher in vegetables, fruits, legumes, and minimally processed grains.

I knew that, and I'm guessing you do, too. Yet the idea of becoming a full-time vegan was neither realistic nor appealing to someone accustomed to eating as widely and as well as I do. Furthermore, I had no interest in becoming an isolated vegan in a world of omnivores and—though I have vegan friends, to be sure—the world of omnivores is where I live. Full time.

Yes. I like vegetables and grains; I love them. I love tofu, too, when prepared well. Even back then, I was eating beans far more frequently than I ever had. But none of this got in the way of my enjoying pork shoulder, pizza, bacon, and burgers. I was not prepared to give up that kind of food. That sounded untenable and, more importantly, unsustainable for more than a couple of weeks.

So the question became: What could I do with the conflict between what was undoubtedly Sid's very sound advice—"become a vegan"—and my own established, beloved, well-socialized lifestyle?

The answer, to me, was this: I'd become a part-time vegan. And for me, this part-time veganism would follow these simple rules: From the time I woke up in the morning until 6 in the evening, I'd eat a super-strict vegan diet, with no animal products at all.

In fact, I decided to go even beyond that: Until 6 P.M., I'd also forgo hyper-processed food, like white bread, white rice, white pasta, of course all junk food, and alcohol.

At 6 P.M., I'd become a free man, allowing myself to eat whatever I wanted, usually—but not always—in moderation. Some nights, this meant a steak dinner; some nights, it was a blow-out meal at a good restaurant; other nights, dinner was a tunafish sandwich followed by some cookies. It ran, and runs, the gamut.

Whatever happened at dinner, though, the next morning I turned not to bacon and eggs or a bowl of Trix but to oatmeal or fruit or vegetables. For lunch, rice and beans or a salad—or both. Throughout the day I snacked on nuts and more fruit.

I called the diet "vegan before six," or VB6. And it worked.

A month later, I weighed myself; I'd lost 15 pounds. A month after that, I went to the lab for blood work: Both my cholesterol and my blood sugar levels were down, well into the normal range (my cholesterol had gone from 240 to 180). My apnea was gone; in fact, for the first time in probably thirty years, I was sleeping through the night, not even snoring. Within four months, I'd lost more than 35 pounds and was below 180—less than I'd weighed in thirty years. And the funny thing was, the way I ate in the daytime began to change the way I ate at night.

So why be vegan just until 6 o'clock? Am I suggesting that 6 P.M. is some kind of magical metabolic witching hour? Not at all. Truthfully, the hour itself doesn't matter much, and if you habitually eat dinner very early, your plan may be VB5—or VB9, if you live in Spain. The point I was making to myself, and that I'm saying to you, is that dinnertime sets you free. Dinnertime, because that's when you're likely to want to eat the most, because that's when you're most likely to drink (and lose discipline!), because that's when you're most likely to combine eating with socializing, an important and even beneficial thing.

But even though the time itself is arbitrary, it has the power to make you stop and think before acting. In fact, the rules are what VB6 has in common with "regular" diets; because anyone can say (and many people do), "Eat sensibly, don't overeat, increase your consumption of fruits and vegetables, eat less junk and high-calorie, low-nutrition foods." If it were that easy, there'd be no need for diets. But by telling you "Don't eat animal products or refined foods during the day, and feel free to eat what you like at night," VB6 gives you the structure you need to exercise limited but effective discipline in a way that accomplishes all of those things.

During the day you'll be observant, and eat way more fruits and vegetables than you probably have until now, and virtually none of the foods that we know cause your metabolism to go haywire, putting a downward spiral in motion. In the evening, you'll still eat more thoughtfully, but won't necessarily avoid or limit foods you love and can't imagine eliminating from your diet. Simply put, at 6 o'clock you can put "the diet" on hold—a compromise that offers the benefits of restraint without the hardship of perpetual denial. Even reading this now, six years after I began, it still sounds pretty good to me.

This is not to say that my adapting to VB6 was seamless. I wasn't exactly "becoming a vegan," but this new diet was certainly not the way I was used to getting through the day. In 2007, when I first embarked on this plan, I'd been a professional food writer (and eater!) for more than twenty-five years. My diet had become increasingly indulgent and untamed, and my opportunities for eating "well"—that is, lavishly— were near constant. I had few rules and, I thought, little need for them. Like many of us, I ate what tasted good to me.

Even before this conversation with Sid, my thinking about food and eating had begun to change—enough so that his suggestion that I become vegan wasn't completely out of left field. I knew, for example, that we Americans eat too much junk food and too many animal products. I knew that food was being produced in an increasingly mechanized and unprincipled manner, without taking into account the welfare of consumers—that's us—or the environment or animals or the people who grew or processed it. And I knew that our health as a country was going down the tubes, and that the Standard American Diet (SAD for short, and it is just that) was at least in part responsible.

The combination of thinking that way and my new way of eating led to profound changes in my life; it changed not only my diet but my work. I didn't want to become a preacher or even a teacher, but the more I thought about our diet, the more I practiced VB6, the more I recognized that these changes were essential not only for our health but for that of the planet and many of the things living on it.

I began to write not only about cooking but about eating, about *food*. I began speaking publicly about the relationships among eating, health, and the environment, and I began changing my work at the *New York Times*: After nearly twenty years of writing about recipes, cooking, and the delights of food, mostly for the Dining section, I branched out to Week In Review and other sections. This led, eventually, to my becoming a *Times* Opinion writer, with my main subject being food: how, what, and why we eat, and the forces that affect those things.

There's no lack of subject matter, that's for sure: Food touches everything. You can't discuss it without considering the environment, health, the role of animals other than humans in this world, the economy, politics, trade, globalization, or most other important issues. This includes such unlikely and seemingly unrelated matters as global warming: Industrialized livestock production, for example, appears to be accountable for a fifth or more of the greenhouse gases that are causing climate change.

But chances are you didn't buy this book to save the planet, or to improve animal welfare, or even to think about those things. You probably bought this book because you wanted to improve your own health or, even more specifically, because you wanted to lose weight.

If that's the case, you've come to the right place, because VB6 can help you do both of those things. My own weight has stabilized and my health has improved over the course of the last six years, and VB6 can do the same for you and help you to do it, not with some two-week snake-oil miracle cure—though you'll probably see changes for the better in the first two weeks you're on this diet, if you take it seriously— but with an easy-to-make change that you'll want to stick to for the rest of your life. And best of all, you will be able to do just that while eating as well as (or better than) you ever have before, and without denying yourself *any* food you really love.

PART ONE

WEIGHT LOSS AND BETTER LIVING

1
The Diet with a Philosophy

You've bought this book for one or two reasons: You want to lose weight, or you want to improve your overall health. And it's likely not the first "diet" book you've bought. But VB6 is a little different, because it relies on a more classic definition of the word *diet*, one that takes a longer-term view.

That word, *diet*. In the twisted, very much American way the word is generally understood, it's a temporary regimen we adopt to lose weight, for two weeks or two months—rarely any longer. A diet is a short-term sacrifice and, you hope, a quick fix: "I'm going on a diet." This kind of diet is something you start reluctantly but with a great sense of hope. You do it for health, or vanity, or self-confidence—or lack thereof. You hope for quick results so you won't have to suffer on this restrictive regimen for long.

Yet you have probably already learned not to expect lasting results. You know that quick-fix diets fail almost every time; they're exercises in futility. You may lose some weight, but as you return to your "normal" way of eating, you inevitably gain it back. (In fact you may even wind up a little heavier.) You may also subsequently experience a sense of failure, guilt, self-disgust, and a profusion of other negative emotions, feeling you've exhausted all of this effort to wind up in no better shape than you were in the first place. You may even feel you've taken a huge step backward, wallow for a bit, and then—as you probably know all too well—decide to go on yet another diet. (There's more about the dieting cycle starting on page 20.)

WHAT IS VB6?

VB6 is different, and it's more in tune with a different definition of *diet*, the one that comes from the Latin *diaita*, which roughly translates as "manner of living": what we'd call lifestyle.

And that's what we're talking about here. VB6 is not a two-week, starve-yourself-and-lose-20-pounds deal, but a lifelong commitment to your health; not just a temporary change in the way you eat, but a permanent change in the way you live. And there's no hocus-pocus, either. It's not a miracle program you "go on" to reach a specific goal, a short-term diet that you'll abandon when that goal is achieved.

In every way, it's better than a crash course in weight loss: There is no full-time sacrifice and there's plenty of enjoyment. Yes, VB6 favors some foods over others, but it doesn't absolutely forbid any foods. The recipes in Part Two provide nutritional information for those who are interested, but I won't ask you to count calories, points, carbs, or anything else.

Nor will I tell you that you must eat foods that you don't want to eat, or to ignore your body's legitimate cravings and desires, or to stop eating before you're full. I am, after all, someone who has built an entire career on my love of cooking and eating good food. And VB6 is the way I eat now, and have for six years.

There are three very basic aspects to VB6. First, you make a commitment to eat more plant foods—fruit, vegetables, whole grains, beans . . . you know what I'm talking about. Second, you make a commitment to eat fewer animal products and highly processed foods, like white bread. And third, you all but eliminate junk foods, most of which are barely foods in the strict sense of the word anyway. (I say "all but eliminate" because everyone needs to break the rules occasionally.)

With the six simple steps outlined in the coming chapters—commonsense methods for identifying *and indulging* your specific style of eating—plus a meal plan and a repertoire of core recipes you can mix and match as you like, you'll be able to make the simple changes in your diet it takes to convert you to what amounts to a part-time vegan.

For some of you, VB6 will instantly make so much sense you'll start today and never stop. (That's how it worked for me.) For others, it's something that will take a bit of preparation, so that you can start with understanding and confidence. That's fine, too.

Most of all, VB6 is an exciting opportunity for you to change not only the way you buy, cook, and eat food but also the way you *think* about it—all day long. It begins with a rational philosophy about the role nourishment—food—plays in our lives; and out of that philosophy grows a practice that will help you develop a healthy, happy, functional, and permanent new relationship with food. The "side effects" of this new relationship between you and food: better health, weight loss, and even a positive effect on the world around you.

VB6 is also realistic. It acknowledges the erratic, busy nature of our lives, and it acknowledges that we all have "bad days," when convenience trumps everything else. But it also maintains that you can love food that tastes good—and eat a lot of it—while you improve your health. VB6 is so simple and flexible that it can be adjusted to any style of life, any schedule, and any tastes. Really.

AMERICANS EAT UPSIDE DOWN

Everyone knows that there are problems with the way we eat. We've developed a never-before-seen diet, a way of eating based on a modern (but already outdated) way of living. We eat unprecedented amounts of refined carbohydrates, especially sugar and hyper-processed flour; fats, usually of all the wrong kinds; and meat and dairy, little of which is produced under decent, let alone ideal, conditions, and which in any case is good for us only in small amounts.

These are the foods that give us the vast majority of calories and, generally speaking, they're precisely the foods we should be eating the least of; it's as if our diet is upside down. (This is why almost any diet that takes us away from the Standard American Diet is an improvement.) Our diet—our manner of eating—is not only unhealthy, as has been well documented; it's also unnatural.

And as odd as VB6 might sound to you at first, it's based on thousands of years of tradition and reflects the way we're meant to eat: a diet composed largely of unprocessed plants, with everything else—including meat—considered a treat. Think of the time before industrial agriculture, or even the hunter-gatherers: Humans ate largely what they found or grew, and if they could kill an animal and eat it, great. In other words, plants were the basis for sustenance, and everything else was opportunistic. Only now, with industrial production of meat and hyper-processed foods, the opportunities to eat non-plant foods have become overwhelming, especially given that we're hardwired to consume once hard-to-find fat and sugar. These changes happened slowly. But because they've also happened exponentially, we've reached the point where our diet is a disaster that threatens human health.

VB6 turns the Standard American Diet right side up with a science-based approach that will make perfect sense to you once you read about it. It's also a philosophy.

When I was developing VB6, I thought a lot about what I wanted it to accomplish. Weight loss, of course, was up there, but it's not the exclusive goal: I wanted good health to be even more important. You can be 10, 20 pounds overweight and still be in great health, and you can be 10, 20 pounds "underweight" and abuse the hell out of your body. (Take, for example, the "cigarette diet." You'd lose weight, as many models can tell you.) And I wanted more than that: I wanted VB6 to bring about a real change, not just a temporary one. I wanted it to demonstrate a personal commitment to changing a broken food system, one that unnecessarily damages the environment, animals, and people. And I wanted it to be pleasurable.

VB6 is all of those things. Like any change, it requires some recalibration, especially if you're currently living on frozen pizza, cheeseburgers, and nachos. But the pleasure of eating *real*, well-prepared food is way deeper than the pleasure of eating a corn-syrup–packed processed snack from a package. (I think you'll be surprised how quickly you'll lose your taste for this stuff anyway, and if you absolutely must have a bag of potato chips, well . . . nothing's stopping you.) And the rewards of spending time in the kitchen with family and friends, cooking a meal from scratch, and then serving that meal to your loved ones, is of far greater value than the ease and convenience of fast, frozen, or junk food. VB6 honors and celebrates the venerable, storied, fulfilling pleasures that food has always brought to humans, a treasured past we're on the verge of losing forever.

A DIET YOU CAN STICK TO

Once you learn the principles and identify your goals and challenges, VB6 can be followed in a way that suits every personality and situation. You'll start with a 28-Day Plan and some recipes (pages 119 and 123), but you'll find that VB6 soon becomes second nature and you won't *need* a plan anymore. And you can't really fail: You might have meals, days, weeks, or even months in which you're not following the principles laid out in this book as closely as you could. (I sure do, if that makes you feel any better.) And you'll certainly have treats and indulgences, as well as desperate moments in which you'll eat whatever is convenient, regardless of where it came from or whether it's good for you. (I do that, too.)

All of that's okay, at least in the short run, because this isn't an approach that aims for perfection; it isn't even especially strict. It's about doing your best to nourish yourself with real, wholesome foods most of the time and not beating yourself up when you don't. As long as you're committed to that, the occasional trip-up is not a big deal.

But I'm betting that VB6 will inspire you to make the changes described in the book and stay dedicated to these new habits because you'll genuinely enjoy the food you're eating. Once you battle through your habitual eating patterns—whether heavy on junk food, animal products, hyper-processed carbs, or all three—you'll find that the rewards of eating real food far exceed those of eating the food that attacks your health. As I said, it's not deprivation: It's substituting new rewards, genuine rewards, for those false rewards that come from a near-addiction for the food that marketers spend billions convincing you to eat.

That's why VB6 works.

Although some people will plunge into VB6-style eating without skipping a beat, most will find meal plans and recipes to be helpful examples, at least at the beginning. The sixty-plus recipes and variations here (which begin on page 136) are, naturally, vegan for breakfast, lunch, and snacks, and include a wide variety of non-vegan ingredients for dinner. They also offer a range of possible options, substitutions, and variations. And if maximizing weight loss is your initial goal, you can adjust the plan, including the portion sizes of the recipes, to reach it more quickly.

The plan and recipes have another role: They offer lifelong eating lessons, along with ways to approach different (and perhaps, to you, new) types of foods. They'll show you which ingredients or categories you can eat in unlimited (truly!) amounts, which you should approach with moderation, and which should be considered treats.

But let me repeat: You don't have to count calories or anything else unless you want to, and if you've ever been on a "regular" diet, or even read about one, you know that's unusual. Most diets have you counting calories, grams of fat, carbohydrates, or points assigned to foods based on their caloric content. All of this turns eating into a clinical exercise and encourages obsessive behavior. And there are two big problems with this kind of dieting, problems I've addressed in conceiving VB6.

For one thing, eating loses its pleasure when food is reduced to a number or a point. Who is going to research, write down, and add up calories for the rest of his or her life? Almost no one. And calorie counting will not only make you miserable; it's not sustainable, and because of that, probably won't be able to keep the weight you lose off for the long haul.

VB6 is simple, flexible, and remarkably easy to maintain. You won't be counting or weighing anything; you'll just be eating the basic food groups in different proportions than you have been: the right proportions. VB6 focuses on the kinds of foods that are good for your body and will help you understand the quantities—and qualities—of foods that help promote weight loss and a lifetime of good health.

Good health is not about weight; weight is an indicator of good health. (Similarly, good health is not about, for example, cholesterol; lower cholesterol is an indicator of good health.) VB6 is not primarily about being skinny but about being *healthy,* and healthy people are, generally speaking, not overweight. Eat a real, practical, sustainable diet, and you'll look and feel terrific. That's the basis of VB6.

WHY WE NEED CHANGE

Being overweight tends to make us sick, and as a nation we are consistently overweight. As a result, the annual obesity-related health-care bill is $150 billion (at least; some estimates are much higher). And it's climbing.

This is why almost any diet that offers a chance to evolve from the status quo, from eating like a caveman to going vegan, represents a vast improvement over the junk-and-meat–laden Standard American Diet (from here on out dubbed SAD). By junk I mean food that either contains no nutritious value whatsoever—like soda—or foods that are loaded with chemicals and so highly processed that even though they might contain some nutritional value, they bear little resemblance to their origins. Some people call these calories "empty," but that makes them sound benign. In fact, they're worse than that; they're harmful.

Incredibly, tellingly, more than half of the calories consumed in America come from junk like soda and doughnuts, hyper-processed foods like white bread, and the products of industrially raised animals.

Why the SAD is so damaging is complicated, as you'll see in a bit. But the processed-food industry makes dietary change a huge challenge by heavily marketing precisely those highly processed sugar- and fat-laden foods that are most harmful—and most profitable. They want us to overconsume that stuff, and we comply.

WHAT WE EAT AND WHY

Some facts and figures: Sweets and desserts account for 12 percent of Americans' daily caloric intake, with soft drinks making up an additional 7 percent (we each drink about 57 gallons of soft drinks annually, or about a pint a day), and we eat an average of 46 slices (23 pounds) of pizza a year.

But here's the capper: Each year, the average American consumes more than 200 pounds of meat and poultry, something like three times the global average (and about 8 ounces a day); and 607 pounds of milk, cheese, and other dairy products. We also eat about 79 pounds of fat a year, a whopping 22 pounds more than we ate in 1980. (The only glimmer of good news here is that we're each eating 10 fewer pounds of shortening and margarine than we were several years ago; both are primary sources of hydrogenated vegetable oil, aka trans fat, a danger to heart health.)

All of that crowds out what we should be eating. We eat 20 percent fewer salads than we did twenty-five years ago, and only one in four meals contain an unprocessed vegetable. (That statistic would be even more dire if the lettuce on a hamburger were not counted as an unprocessed vegetable.) Only 49 percent of Americans ate a salad (just one!) in the last two weeks. *Maybe* 10 percent of our calories come from the unprocessed fruits and vegetables that should be the source of *most* of our calories.

The result is illness. Never before have our waistlines been so wide and our rates of diabetes so high, and the correlation between the two is undisputed. Two-thirds of Americans are overweight, and more than one-third of adults (35.7%)—upward of 72 million people—are obese. Seventeen percent of children are also obese. (Obesity rates for adults have doubled since 1980; for children, they've *tripled*.)

Scary enough, but perhaps even more staggering are the results of a study finding that 70 percent of obese children have at least one risk factor for cardiovascular disease, while 39 percent have two risk factors. We have reached a point where children are exhibiting signs of diseases that were once reserved for those in middle age.

Why are we doing this?

Part of it is physical: Some studies indicate that highly processed foods might literally be addictive. (In part this is because we're hardwired to eat sugar and fat; we need them both to live, just not in the forms and quantities we're getting them now.) Most of us eat around the holes in our busy schedules, and it's difficult to get away from the habit of eating ubiquitous, "convenient" junk. And sometimes we eat to satisfy emotional cravings or out of boredom.

But for the most part we are victims of the most successful marketing campaign in history: More than $11 billion is spent each year promising everything from flavor to health to happiness, almost all in the name of processed foods, and more than $4 billion is spent by the fast-food industry alone. All of these factors fuel the obesity pandemic.

THE COSTS OF THE STANDARD AMERICAN DIET

This marketing comes at a price. It's expensive to be sick, and obesity cripples not only our personal health but also our health-care system and even our economy. As I mentioned, the economic costs are mind-boggling: $150 billion a year, and climbing. (It's predicted to reach 18 percent of total health-care spending in the next twenty years or so.)

At a time in history when the government is fiscally strapped and struggles to find money not only for school lunches but also for schools, spending money on *preventable* health issues caused by easily changed eating habits is unfortunate, to say the least. If but a portion of the money that goes to subsidize the production of junk were instead used to encourage a diet of real food, the changes would be dramatic.

But the SAD wreaks havoc on way more than health-care costs: It degrades the environment, arguably an even bigger issue than obesity-related disease. The industrial production of animal products and hyper-processed food creates devastating by-products, from greenhouse gas emissions to land degradation to polluted water supplies.

It's commonly acknowledged that livestock production is one of the top two contributors to greenhouse gas emissions, accounting for at least 20 percent (and by some estimates up to 50 percent) of dangerous gases in the atmosphere—a greater impact than even transportation.

Give that a minute to sink in: Growing animals for food in an industrial fashion is worse for the environment than almost anything else humans have figured out how to do, including driving cars.

I could go on about the pollutants, water and land use, antibiotics (80% of antibiotics in the U.S. go to livestock, and you've undoubtedly heard about the problems that causes), hormones, fertilizers, pesticides, and erosion—but you get the point.

These problems will worsen as long as high consumption of cheap meat and industrialized production continue. We'll have to raise a staggering 120 billion animals a year by 2050 just to meet demand at the current levels; and this, obviously, is unsustainable. The only solution is to reduce demand and therefore production.

Processed foods are also environmental culprits. Raising, manufacturing, storing, and transporting food accounts for 10 percent of all fossil-fuel use in the United States—about the same as France's total energy consumption. Consider that a single can of soda (which offers about 150 nutrient-free calories) requires 2,200 calories of energy to produce, while the aluminum tray that holds a TV dinner takes nearly 1,500 calories to make. All food requires some energy to grow or be produced, but production accounts for only about 20 percent of our food-related energy consumption; the rest is associated with processing, freezing, packaging, and so on. This means that highly processed foods take a much higher toll on the environment.

Then there are moral issues: We need the "efficiency" of large-scale industrial animal factories to satisfy our current needs, and this production means we're torturing the billions of animals we produce each year. As you probably know, animals grown in factory farms live in horrific conditions; they're kept in cages or pens so tiny that they don't have room to turn around, and they're drugged, mutilated, and denied the opportunity to fulfill every natural instinct they have. Again, I could go on.

Don't get me wrong: Like more than 95 percent of the people in the United States, I'm a meat-eater. But the way most animals are raised in the United States is appalling, and I don't think anyone with a conscience could disagree with me. The only way to change this is to eat less meat. And that's an integral part of VB6.

"CONVENIENCE" IS KILLING US

Virtually every product we put in our mouths is sold by one of only ten multi-national companies, and the financial and political power of Big Food is impossible to overstate: During the last couple of decades well over a hundred billion dollars has been spent convincing us to choose so-called convenience food over real food. (In the U.S. almost $1 billion a year is spent selling soda alone.) And the corporations have big help: Government subsidies that make it easier and more profitable to grow and process the ingredients in junk have helped determine our food choices for decades. In fact, if so-called specialty crops (that's what the Department of Agriculture calls fruits and vegetables) were subsidized the same way that corn and soybeans are, the American food landscape would look entirely different.

Of course preparing real food takes time. And admittedly, not everyone wants to or is even able to allocate time to cook. Yet the marketing of convenience food was largely responsible for the near death of home cooking, which in turn has affected not only our health but our attitudes about cooking and eating. The future looks even more grim: Big Food now spends about $1.6 billion a year to sell this food to children under the age of 17 in an attempt to make our dreadful diet permanent.

It doesn't help that Big Macs—or whatever your junk food of choice might be—aren't just convenient, they're super-convenient. Their perpetual availability fuels a cycle of reckless indulgence by making it easy to eat inexpensive, often harmful meals at any time of day or night, without even leaving your car.

Big Food also hawks convenience to people trying to make healthier food choices or lose weight. Labeling and marketing something as "fat-free" or "heart-healthy," or touting a specific nutrient like fiber, gives the unmistakable impression that these products have fewer calories or that the claimed benefits are somehow better than eating a less processed version of the same food. And it works: $40 billion is spent a year on weight-loss diets and products. (That's about 7 percent of the $538 billion prepared food industry.)

For example, take a look at a "healthy" "diet" bar, which is nothing more than junk food marketed as diet food. (And this isn't a trick; there are dozens if not hundreds of similar examples.)

And it isn't just mock candy bars that lay traps for would-be dieters. Take a look at a couple of typical diet "lunches" that you might bring to the office, and compare them to a lunch recipe from this book. Start with the almost incredible difference in ingredients, inevitable since the home-cooked meal requires only real food. The VB6 soup is about twice as big a portion, but only 30 percent more calories, without any of the cholesterol and hardly any sugar, with none of it added sugar. Yet the protein is on par, even though the meal contains no animal foods. And the soup has either five or ten times more fiber, depending on which frozen entrée you choose.

You might also think that 0-calorie sodas and handy 100-calorie snack packs would help us slim down, but the opposite is true: These marketing ploys with their nonsensical health claims are a central part of the problem. The idea of special diets to counter the effects of our

Diet Bar vs. Candy Bar

PRODUCT	SLIM-FAST SWEET AND SALTY CHOCOLATE ALMOND BAR (45G)	KIT KAT BAR (45G)
CALORIES	200	230
FAT	8g	12g
SODIUM	190mg	35mg
CARBOHYDRATES	23g	29g
PROTEIN	9g	3g

INGREDIENTS (SLIM-FAST BAR): Soy crisp with cocoa (soy protein isolate, tapioca starch, cocoa [processed with alkali], calcium carbonate), almonds, fructose, dry roasted peanuts, chocolate-flavored coating (sugar, fractionated palm kernel oil, cocoa [processed with alkali], lactose, dextrose, soy lecithin, natural flavor, partially hydrogenated palm oil), polydextrose, enriched wheat flour (wheat flour, niacin, iron, thiamin mononitrate, riboflavin, folic acid), toasted rolled oats (rolled oats, high fructose corn syrup, soybean oil, honey), corn syrup, milk, water, cocoa (processed with alkali), glycerin, inulin, chocolate, sunflower oil, maltodextrin, butter (cream, salt), palm oil, nonfat milk, sugar, salt, fractionated palm kernel oil, natural and artificial flavor, soy lecithin, whey, locust bean gum, sucralose and acesulfame potassium (nonnutritive sweeteners), dextrose, nonfat yogurt powder (cultured nonfat milk), sodium bicarbonate, mixed tocopherols (used to protect quality), artificial color, partially hydrogenated palm oil, soybean oil, gum arabic, brown sugar, citric acid, caramel color. Vitamins and minerals: calcium carbonate, potassium chloride, ascorbic acid, vitamin E acetate, niacinamide, biotin, folic acid, pyridoxine hydrochloride (vitamin B_6), riboflavin, vitamin A palmitate, calcium pantothenate, cyanocobalamin (vitamin B_{12}), thiamin mononitrate, phytonadione (vitamin K1), cholecalciferol (vitamin D_3). Contains milk, peanuts, soy, wheat, and almonds. May contain eggs, sesame, cashews, coconut, pecans, and walnuts.

INGREDIENTS (KIT KAT BAR): Milk chocolate (sugar, modified milk ingredients, cocoa butter, unsweetened chocolate, lactose, soya lecithin, polyglycerol polyricinoleate, artificial flavor), wheat flour, sugar, hydrogenated soybean oil or modified palm oil, unsweetened chocolate, sodium bicarbonate, soya lecithin, yeast, artificial flavor.

SOURCES: UNILEVER/SLIM FAST AND NESTLÉ/KIT KAT PRODUCT INFORMATION.

day-to-day eating habits, the SAD, is a recent phenomenon, which makes sense: So is mass obesity. The SAD has essentially created the need for weight-loss diets, and the two go hand in hand.

In fact, the SAD is best described as a vicious cycle of consuming hyper-processed, brilliantly marketed junk along with the diet schemes intended to combat the very system they're a part of. We've been taught to label food as "good" and "bad"—we first consume more of the bad, and then we turn to dieting as a salve. But not only does deprivational dieting not work, it serves to further pathologize eating, turning food into the enemy and celebrating a weird kind of perverse asceticism. And this anxiety can turn a natural, normal, and enjoyable activity into something largely negative.

No matter what the marketing says, hyper-processed convenience

Frozen Diet Lunch vs. VB6 Lunch

ENTRÉE	LEAN CUISINE CHICKEN FRIED RICE (9 OUNCES)	LEAN CUISINE BEEF AND BROCCOLI (9 OUNCES)	GREENS AND BEANS SOUP (ABOUT 18 OUNCES; PAGE 164)
CALORIES	260	270	384
FAT	5g	5g	9g
SODIUM	530mg	520mg	567mg
CHOLESTEROL	25g	20g	0g
CARBOHYDRATES	41g	43g	62g
FIBER	4g	2g	21g
SUGARS	5g	9g	1g
PROTEIN	12g	12g	20g

INGREDIENTS (LEAN CUISINE CHICKEN FRIED RICE): Blanched enriched long-grain parboiled rice (water, rice, iron, niacin, thiamin mononitrate, folic acid), cooked white meat chicken (white meat chicken, water, modified tapioca starch, chicken flavor [dried chicken broth, chicken powder, natural flavor], carrageenan, whey protein concentrate, soybean oil, corn syrup solids, sodium phosphate, salt), water, carrots, peas, soy sauce (water, wheat, soybeans, salt), green onions, 2% or less of onions, modified cornstarch, sesame oil, brown sugar, soybean oil, garlic puree, white vinegar, brown sugar syrup, ginger puree (ginger, water, citric acid), sugar, yeast extract, potassium chloride, caramel color, dehydrated red peppers, lactic acid, spice, calcium lactate, smoke flavoring.

INGREDIENTS (LEAN CUISINE BEEF AND BROCCOLI): Blanched enriched long-grain parboiled rice (water, rice, iron, niacin, thiamin mononitrate, folic acid), water, seasoned cooked beef product (beef, water, dextrose, modified cornstarch, potassium chloride, salt, sodium and potassium phosphates, caramel color, natural flavors), broccoli, water chestnuts, brown sugar, 2% or less of rice wine vinegar, soy sauce (water, wheat, soybeans, salt), green onions, hoisin sauce (sugar, water, sweet potatoes, salt, modified cornstarch, soybeans, spices, sesame seeds, wheat flour, garlic, chili pepper, acetic acid), carrots, yellow carrots, modified cornstarch, garlic puree, sesame seeds, sesame oil, sugar, chicken broth, soybean oil, potassium chloride, chili garlic sauce (salted chili peppers [chili peppers, salt], garlic, sugar, rice vinegar, water, modified cornstarch, acetic acid), yeast extract, dehydrated soy sauce (soybeans, salt, wheat), caramel color, spice, citric acid.

INGREDIENTS (GREENS AND BEANS SOUP): Greens (collards, broccoli rabe, or escarole), dried beans (like white beans), water, onion, olive oil, garlic, salt, black pepper.

SOURCES: NESTLÉ/LEAN CUISINE PRODUCT INFORMATION; CALCULATED FROM THE USDA NATIONAL NUTRIENT DATABASE FOR STANDARD REFERENCE.

foods can't possibly be as nourishing as real food. But again, the very goal of marketing is to confound and mislead us on this key point. We're taught to worry about the things that make food bad, like fat, sugar, and salt, and to eat food that contains "good" things, like protein. Therefore, meat is "good" because it's high in protein; breakfast cereal is "healthy" because it's fortified with fiber and vitamins.

But isolating nutrients enables Big Food to take its hyper-processed junk, load it up with fiber, contend that it's low-salt or low-fat, and sell it to you as healthy. Not only is this nonsense, it makes everyday eating far more complicated than it needs to be; a healthy diet is nothing more than a variety of minimally processed foods.

WHY MOST DIETS DON'T WORK

The Standard American Diet—SAD—got us into this mess, and although we need action on the part of both government and corporations to change production methods and limit marketing, none of us can afford to wait for change to come from above: We all have to begin to change the way we eat.

Start by asking yourself, Do you want a quick fix to lose weight before going back to eating like you did yesterday? Or are you looking for real, meaningful, long-term change, change that will not only take off weight but improve your overall health? Are you reluctant to turn over this new leaf, procrastinating a bit? Or are you excited at the prospect of taking your life in a different direction?

COMMITTING TO POSITIVE CHANGE

Whether you start today, next week, or next month, it's important to see that changing how you eat—which is what VB6 will do—is not a temporary detour. It's a new road, a better road, and the road we're meant to be on, one that emphasizes real, natural (sorry, but there's no better word) foods and that treats the dominant foods of the SAD as once-in-a-while things. The goal of VB6 is to improve your overall health: how you feel, how you look, how you live. And—no question—that will take some discipline, especially at first. But unlike other diets, VB6 is not a short-term fix but a lifestyle change that's designed to inspire new habits by exploring the pleasures and benefits of real food.

Most weight-loss diets refuse to strike a balance, demonizing either carbs or fats or specific foods. On such restrictive programs, it's no wonder that many people can lose weight for a short period of time but few can keep weight off long term. Only one in six overweight and obese adults report having maintained weight loss of at least 10 percent for one year. Even more short term than that: The average weight-loss attempt is four weeks for women, six weeks for men. Clearly most modern diets are promoting short-term solutions to a lifelong problem.

And they fail precisely because they're short-term. We think of them as plans, programs, or protocols—things that we suffer for a period of time in order to reach a goal: Lose XX pounds. But the best prescriptive diets focus on these questions: What will I do once I've reached my goal, once I've lost the weight? How will I keep it off and live a normal life? And that's the most important issue you need to focus on. Because there are definitely diets that will cause you to lose weight faster than VB6. There are not, however, diets that will allow you to live a better life, long-term.

There isn't much future when you tether your diet to the SAD. Plugging baked potato chips or low-fat cream cheese into your diet theoretically reduces your caloric intake, but in reality you're likely to eat more of the low-fat stuff and pile on the calories anyway, and you're still not eating very well. Even if you do manage to lose weight, almost inevitably it will all creep back—and then some—leaving you with a sense of failure, guilt, self-disgust, frustration, and incomprehension at why the diet didn't "work." So you go back to the SAD. And after a while you decide to go on another diet. It's a vicious cycle.

FEAR OF FOOD

Predictably if unfortunately, most diet companies—and most diet books, for that matter—have a vested interest in maintaining the status quo of our diet-obsessed culture and in promoting overly strict, unhealthy diets that are bound to fail. They encourage the SAD vicious cycle through an unrealistic, unnatural way of eating that includes cutting out entire food groups; obsessively counting calories; plugging in unsatisfying, bland "diet" junk for "regular" junk; and in general ignoring our bodies' signals. They encourage a fundamentally unsustainable and often unpleasant way of eating, with a strict or stringent program, plan, or protocol that dictates exactly what we eat, when, and how much.

And that's how they stay in business: by making sure that their product or concept *doesn't work over the long haul*; their profit models rely on people falling off the wagon and finding their way back on, over and over again. The schemes and books proliferate simply because most diets eventually fail. (I'm aware that every diet book says "this is the one that works, and the others are shams." But there's no way around my saying it, too. And what makes VB6 different is that it's a pleasurable and sustainable lifelong plan.)

Many diets eliminate certain types of foods: sugars, starches, fats, or animal products. And of course they work in the short term; it's easy to lose weight when you cut out an entire category of foods, like carbohydrates. Nor is it a wonder that they fail in the long term: It's hard not to feel deprived when you cut out an entire category of foods. (At their worst, you're asked to survive primarily on cabbage soup for weeks at a time.)

Diets also fail because we enjoy eating and require a variety of food to feel satisfied; we're not cut out for a life of self-denial and monotony. Unfortunately, the attitudes that diets beat into us stick around even after the diets have gone south. I know few people who don't have unpleasant emotions surrounding food, who don't feel guilty about overindulging or eating a rich dessert, despite the fact that these are normal occasional activities. It's daily overindulgence—whether in desserts or anything else—that isn't normal, and that's what most diets fail to change in the long run.

To make matters worse, many diets bury you in data, requiring you to count calories, points, or grams of fats or carbohydrates. Counting calories can of course be an effective dieting strategy; if you consume fewer calories than you burn, you'll lose weight. But it turns eating into a clinical, obsessive exercise, reduces food to numbers, eliminates pleasure, and makes the diet unsustainable. No one wants to count calories his or her whole life, while all the time following a program that eliminates huge groups of foods.

The primary example of this type of diet is the enduring low-carb craze (Atkins lives!). Low-carb diets help you shed pounds quickly because your body burns carbohydrates before it burns fat, so if you eliminate bread, pasta, grains, and even many fruits and vegetables from your diet, your body will start burning fat directly.

Two problems arise, however: First, not many people can go their whole lives without eating a banana. (Nor should they.) This diet is as hard on your mind as it is on your body.

Which brings us to the second point: There are serious health risks associated with cutting out entire groups of foods. A recent peer-reviewed study published in the *Journal of the American Medical Association* (that is, an utterly credible study) compared weight loss on three diets: low-fat, low-glycemic (a way to measure blood sugar described in detail on page 47), and low-carb. All participants were allowed the same number of calories. When people were put on the low-carb diet, they burned about 350 calories a day more than those on the low-fat diet, even though they were consuming the same number of calories. A low-glycemic diet had an intermediate effect: The participants burned about 150 calories more than on the low-fat diet.

Sounds clear-cut, right? A low-carb diet is the best way to drop weight.

But if you look more closely, you see that the low-fat diet was flawed from the get-go, since it allowed for processed carbohydrates—the kind found in packaged snacks, for example—which not only contribute to weight gain but are, on the whole, close to non-food.

And the differences between the low-glycemic and low-carb diets are even more revealing. The study found that strictly limiting carbohydrates while emphasizing animal protein raised the levels of cortisol and C-reactive protein (CRP) in the blood; both of these hormones induce stress and inflammation. (High cortisol is believed to promote obesity, insulin resistance, and cardiovascular diseases.)

So not only is low-carb difficult to maintain because it restricts one large and necessary category of food (carbs provide fiber and nutrients not found elsewhere), it also encourages the consumption of animal products in unhealthful quantities, and has scary and undesirable physical effects. Beyond those mentioned above, it induces ketosis, a form of starvation that is not only unpleasant but dangerous. Start eating carbs and these problems go away . . . and the pounds come back.

That's why low-carb diets are no more than quick fixes, and the same has invariably been found true of any other diet that requires us to severely limit a whole group of macronutrients—carbohydrates, protein, or fat—or avoid them all together. In the long run, your body and mind don't do well with this kind of deprivation.

Back to the study: It's interesting that the low-glycemic (low-sugar) diet promoted *sustained* and consistent weight-loss maintenance without any major restrictions. (Of all the weight-loss regimens that have been studied by major, credible institutions, it's the diet most similar to VB6.) Of the three diets, it came out best in the study, providing steady, if somewhat slower, and sustained weight loss without requiring a bizarre diet and without negative effects.

Of course, some conventional dietary strategies work. Dieters who keep food diaries are generally more successful at losing weight and keeping it off than those who don't. As with any form of learning, writing can help etch the lesson in your memory, and logging heightens awareness.

This explains the ongoing success of the Weight Watchers program, which is consistently reported by its users and others as the easiest diet to follow and maintain over long periods of time. (In fact, much of Weight Watchers—including the social aspect, the friendly attitude toward real fruits and vegetables, and the good recipes—makes a great deal of sense. But the program supports the nation's junk-food habit by promoting hyper-processed snacks and "diet" foods, from which they profit mightily.)

Other studies have shown that financial incentives work for some people: Dangling cash as a carrot helped participants stay on a diet, and men who bet they'd lose weight fared better than those who didn't. So if you think getting your friends to join in some kind of VB6 challenge will help you in your endeavor to get healthier, by all means ask them. Do whatever it takes to replace old habits with new ones.

But you don't need help to go VB6 (and I won't pay you!); you need only a commitment to refrain from animal products and hyper-processed foods until dinnertime. This is not insignificant or without challenges, but again I can say that for me and many others, it's a sustainable endeavor that becomes easier over time.

2

Why VB6 *Does* Work

Knowing how VB6 works will give you more patience with and belief in the process. It's not hard to understand, and it's based on well-established, fundamental principles.

It begins, of course, with the calorie—a measurement of energy, nothing more or less—and how the calories in carbohydrates, protein, and fat function in the body.

Calories matter, of course, but the truth is that if you change your diet to favor plants, you're almost guaranteed—without thinking, or at least without obsessing—to consume fewer calories than you did when you were eating the Standard American Diet (SAD). In the SAD, more than a quarter of the calories come from highly processed and damaging carbohydrates, like soda and doughnuts, and another quarter come from animal products. When you're VB6, you'll be getting a majority of your calories from unprocessed plant foods, and plants have fewer calories relative to their weight—that is, they have a lower *caloric density*. (We could call this calorie density—which I prefer—or energy density, too; they're all equivalent terms.)

THE CONVERSION OF FOOD TO ENERGY

The concept of burning energy is directly related to how you lose weight—or don't. Knowing a little about how the calories in carbohydrates, proteins, and fats are used, or burned, or metabolized, will help you understand why VB6 works.

As I've described, VB6 came about pragmatically, and only in retrospect did I realize that it draws upon four main nutrition themes: One, it recognizes that you don't lose weight without reducing your calorie intake. Two, it sees some categories of foods as nothing more than calorie bombs that should be avoided. Three, it acknowledges that your body treats different foods differently. And four, it asserts that real food is better for you than hyper-processed food, "food" that doesn't even meet the definition of food.

This last factor—the real food factor—is precisely what makes VB6 radically different. Not only will you be changing the way you eat forever, rather than plunging temporarily into a radical diet, you'll be eating what your body needs to work properly and feel its best.

FOOD AS FUEL

Thinking of your body as a machine remains a handy way to explain some of the science of metabolism, the discussion of "calories in, calories out." As with any machine—you might think of a car—your body is a finite system of interdependent parts that must consume energy in order to move, breathe, think, live. And (as you may remember from high school), the laws of thermodynamics state that energy and matter can neither be created nor destroyed, but can only be transformed or converted from one form to another.

So you can turn one kind of energy (chemical, for example) into another (like kinetic), or you can convert energy into matter or matter into energy, but you can't simply summon up either and you can't make either just go away. In the case of our bodies, the energy and matter in food (which come from carbohydrates, protein, and fat, and which is measured in calories) is converted during digestion into both a different form of energy—the fuel we can use to function—and different forms of matter: the material that makes up the bulk of our bodies, our muscles, bones, blood, and so on.

More specifically, metabolism is essentially a series of oxidation processes in which the molecules from protein (amino acids), carbohydrates (sugars), and fat (fatty acids) are either broken down to produce energy or used to replenish our bodily structures. This conversion creates carbon dioxide, water, and waste, which we exhale and secrete and excrete.

Now this is key: When we consume more matter than our body needs, the body first transforms some of it into energy and then converts the remainder to fat. That fat is stored, since our super-efficient machine saves energy for a time when we might need it.

Remember: It's only recently that the majority of humans could pretty much be assured of having enough to eat, so—because evolution works very slowly, at least in the way we perceive it—our bodies still anticipate the "inevitable" famine. Imagine how well that worked when our ancestors lived through weeks or months of real hunger. During those times, when they'd consume less energy than their bodies needed, that stored fat was actually used, transformed to fuel and burned off.

The good news is that relatively few people go through periods of prolonged famine. The bad news is that our bodies don't know that; the evolutionary process hasn't caught up with our current reality. We continue to store excess intake as fat. Not only do we not need that fat but it isn't good for us: It clogs things up and causes problems. Big ones, like diabetes, heart disease, and cancer.

Exactly how much fuel a body needs at any time is sometimes called the "total energy expenditure," which includes what you need to stay alive (the basal metabolic rate, or BMR) and what you need to move around (the energy expenditure of physical activity, or EEPA). Our bodies need a fair amount of fuel just to idle: The BMR usually gobbles up about two-thirds of your daily energy output; the EEPA accounts for the other third. Regulating our body temperature used to burn a lot of calories, too, but these days we regulate external temperature (through heating, air conditioning, and effective clothing) so our machine doesn't work as hard as it once did to stay warm or keep cool. (This is why some wacky contemporary diets include cold baths; if you chill yourself, your body needs to expend energy to stay warm. Probably if you walked around with a hat full of ice cubes, you could burn a few extra calories also.)

You often hear people claiming to have a slow or fast metabolism as a way to explain how what they eat affects their weight. What they're saying is that the rate at which they convert food to fuel is either efficient or inefficient—like a car getting better or worse gas mileage. This analogy might still be a good one, except the variables that control how food is converted to energy and either burned or stored are among the most complex and contested fields of scientific study. So trying to characterize your metabolism as either slow or fast is simplistic at best and—unless you undergo a series of tests to try to determine your specific molecular and hormonal makeup—probably futile or wishful thinking.

At the heart of this process is the calorie, the measure of energy and the mother of points, indexes, loads, densities—all of the ways people keep track of what they put in their mouths. And while VB6 works even if you count nothing, understanding calories will help you understand why it's successful.

THE CALORIE CONUNDRUM

The calorie is the most common way to measure the fuel that runs the body. One calorie represents the amount of energy needed to increase the temperature of 1 gram of water (a little less than ¼ teaspoon) by 1°C at sea level.

That's specific and simple, but determining the number of calories your body needs is not. In fact it's incredibly challenging, because it depends on many variables: physical activity, age, body composition, time of day, stress, sex, hormones, and established weight—just for starters. Recent studies have revealed the role that microbes in our gut play in burning calories; others question the accuracy of the calculations that appear on labels. It's not just math: "I need this much energy, so I should consume this many calories."

Determining how many calories you need is difficult, but the government has made things even more confusing. The Food and Drug Administration (FDA) suggests a healthy diet of 2,000 calories a day on all food labels, but most men and women actually need *more* than that; only the most sedentary and frail people can get by on so few calories. Moderately active women in a more or less normal weight range expend at least 2,400 calories a day; for men, that number climbs above 3,000. But the range is very, very wide, and this is yet another argument against obsessively counting calories: You probably don't know how many is too many—except in retrospect, when you find you've gained weight.

This uncertainty explains why diets that claim to manipulate metabolism are so popular: The idea that you can accelerate how calories are burned has obvious appeal. And, indeed, there's evidence that certain foods eaten at a specific time, or in combination, or in abundance, are digested differently than they might be otherwise. But this research is in its early stages, and not yet convincing, so I've steered VB6 clear of metabolic hocus-pocus, relying instead on well-understood, established metabolic principles.

Although no two of us have identical calorie requirements, what's clear is this: Eat too many more calories than you expend through your basal metabolic rate and physical activity, and you will likely gain weight. Conversely, you can maintain a fairly constant weight by balancing the calories you need and the calories you expend.

You probably eat more calories some days and fewer others, but the key word here is *balance*. In fact, for most people striking this balance isn't so difficult; your weight tends to stabilize over time. However, it may stabilize at a place that you (or your doctor) believes is too high, probably because you established a pattern of consuming too many calories, and eventually your body determined that it wanted to "protect"—that is, maintain—that higher weight. (Why, given the same caloric intake, some people gain more weight than others remains a mystery.) Remember, your body is not easily going to give up that stored fat: It "thinks" you might run out of food at any given moment.

For the purposes of analyzing VB6, and taking into account what we can easily know and control about ourselves, let's agree that for weight maintenance there must be a balance of calories consumed and calories expended, and that we need to consume fewer calories than we expend in order to lose weight.

The science is so young that we can legitimately say only this: If you eat more calories than you need for your energy output, you'll *probably* gain weight; and if you eat fewer calories, you'll *probably* lose it.

But increasingly the research indicates that the *kind* of calories you eat can also help determine whether you lose or gain weight. Because *not all calories are created equal*: Hyper-processed junk foods appear to be "fattening," to use a quaint term. Their calories have a greater negative impact than the calories of real, unprocessed foods. This is debatable (and a hot topic among nutritional researchers), but the evidence is piling up: All calories are *not* the same.

What's simple to understand is that carbohydrates and proteins yield 4 calories per gram; fat yields 9 calories per gram. (Alcohol, if you're wondering, comes in at 7 calories.) Fiber—and this is important—contains 0 calories, as does water. If you consume only fiber and water, you'll die. If, however, you eat lots of fiber and water, you'll not only live, you'll live better. It's almost as simple as that. For the most part, if a food is composed mostly of water and fiber, you can eat more of it; if it contains little water or fiber, you should eat less of it. This brings us back to calorie density.

WHAT IS CALORIE DENSITY?

Calorie density is a measure of how much water, fat, and fiber different foods contain: Foods with more water and/or fiber and less fat have a lower density; the reverse yields higher density. Put another way, calorie density measures the ratio between energy content (which is the same as its calorie count, since calories measure energy) and weight. Most plant foods have few calories relative to their weight because they're high in fiber and water, neither of which contains any calories.

Lettuce, for instance, has a calorie density of 0.1, which means that 1 gram of lettuce contains 0.1 calories. Bacon, by contrast, has a calorie density of 5.4, because 1 gram of bacon contains 5.4 calories. Put in terms of how much you might eat in daily life, 1 ounce (approximately 28g) of bacon, or about one slice, contains 153 calories, or fifty-four times as many calories as 1 ounce of lettuce (about ½ cup), with 2.8 calories. And if you eat, say, six slices of bacon, and 2 cups of lettuce (which is a lot), you're now talking about the difference between 918 calories and about 11 calories. Now—and this is about as basic as VB6 can get—think about a lightly dressed salad for lunch instead of a cheeseburger.

A Taste of Calorie Density

FOOD	CALORIE DENSITY	FOOD	CALORIE DENSITY
Iceberg lettuce	0.14	Whole wheat spaghetti (cooked)	1.24
Celery	0.16	White rice	1.30
Tomatoes	0.18	Black beans (cooked)	1.32
Spinach	0.23	Egg (hard-boiled)	1.55
Gatorade	0.26	White flour spaghetti (cooked)	1.58
Grapefruit	0.32	Fish fillet (bluefish, cooked)	1.59
Strawberries	0.32	Chickpeas (cooked)	1.64
Coca-Cola (12 ounces)	0.32	Chicken breast (cooked)	1.65
Broccoli	0.34	Dried apples	2.43
Carrots	0.41	Commercial whole wheat bread	2.47
Milk (1% fat)	0.42	White bread	2.65
Beets	0.43	Whole wheat flour	3.40
Apple juice	0.46	White flour	3.64
Apples (without skin)	0.48	Special K cereal	3.78
Tofu (firm)	0.70	Pretzels	3.80
Bulgur (cooked)	0.83	Parmesan cheese	3.92
Corn	0.86	Twix	5.02
Sweet potatoes (cooked)	0.90	Bacon (cooked)	5.41
Regular potatoes (cooked)	0.97	Cashews (raw)	5.53
Brown rice (cooked)	1.11	Olive oil	8.84
Lentils (cooked)	1.16	Vegetable oil (grapeseed oil)	8.84
Quinoa (cooked)	1.20		

SOURCE: CALCULATED FROM THE USDA NATIONAL NUTRIENT DATABASE FOR STANDARD REFERENCE.

Let's compare apples to apples: 1 cup of chopped fresh apple has 57 calories, while 1 cup of dried apple slices—from which all the water has been removed—has 209 calories. Calculating the calorie density per gram assigns fresh apples with a super-low count of 0.52 and dried with a moderately high 2.43.

But calorie density alone doesn't explain everything. Because unsweetened apple juice comes in at 114 calories a cup, for a density of 0.46. Since beverages have lots of water and no fat, their density can be low, even though they might not be terribly nutritious. (Even soda and sports drinks have low calorie density.) Apples, for example, have way more fiber than their juice.

There's another obvious flaw with calorie density: Remembering and counting these numbers is as counterproductive as counting calories. (If you're interested, see the nutrient database at http://ndb.nal .usda.gov/. There, you can look up almost all kinds of foods and find the number of calories per 100 grams; just move the decimal over two places to the left to get the calorie density.)

On its own, calorie density is inadequate; it's part of the information we need, but not all of it. Still, it's useful for helping us group foods into categories. I do this in detail later, but let's take a quick look at the calorie density of a handful of foods before moving on. In the next section, I'm going to be comparing this list to the glycemic index, another way of looking at the same foods. And then we'll take a look at how these two lists inform the VB6 principles.

Scroll down the list on page 33, and the pattern should quickly become clear: The more water in a food, the lower the calorie density.

THE TROUBLE WITH (SOME) CARBS

We live in carbohydrate country: According to the Centers for Disease Control, Americans get about 50 percent of their daily calories from foods like soda, bread, pasta, pretzels, fries, oatmeal, and other "carbs." (The quotes are here because no food is pure carb—or protein, or fat, or anything else. Food is complex.) We each eat 140 pounds of potatoes per year, about 1 potato per day, mostly in the form of fries and chips. (Collectively we eat 4.5 billion pounds of fries and 2 billion pounds of chips a year.) And both of these options are fried in enough fat to double the number of calories in the potatoes themselves.

Carbohydrates, like fat and protein, are one of the three major components of food; they're also called macronutrients. We once thought of carbohydrates as benign, and it's easy to see why. Fruits, vegetables, and grains are all largely composed of carbohydrates. But unlike fats and protein (which we'll get to shortly), carbohydrates tend to be low or moderate in their calorie density. In their natural state—as opposed to their processed, fast-food state, a key distinction—they have no added sugar and little or no fat.

But a major problem with the SAD is not the *amount* of carbohydrates we're eating, but the *kind* or, more precisely, the way they're processed and sold. Fruits and vegetables are not a part of the problem; the problem—largely—is hyper-processed grains, a form of food that barely existed 100 years ago. It's the hyper-processing of grains (and, less often, but frequently enough, of fruits and vegetables) that brings us a host of ills, from soda to fries to "snacks" to fluffy white bread.

Thanks in part to the many misguided and misguiding official government dietary guidelines issued in the last fifty years, and an agricultural system based almost entirely on just a handful of crops, we consume more products made from grains than ever before. And, of course, we're not eating mostly brown rice and quinoa, but Frosted Flakes and doughnuts.

Why? Because Big Food makes a lot more money processing corn and wheat into snacks and cereals than they do growing and milling whole grains. When manufacturers take a whole food and mix it with a bunch of fat, salt, sugar, and chemicals to make a snack or other packaged food, it's described as "adding value," even though in fact the value is decreased. Put billions of marketing dollars behind that stuff (which, as I mentioned earlier, is increasingly thought of as addictive), and people will pay more for it than they will for (decreasingly available) real whole grains.

Nor are so-called healthy processed foods a substitute for the real

Wheat Thins vs. Wheat Berries

	1 RECOMMENDED SERVING WHEAT THINS ("ORIGINAL BAKED"; ABOUT 1 OUNCE)	½ CUP COOKED WHEAT BERRIES (HARD RED WINTER WHEAT; ABOUT 3.5 OUNCES)
CALORIES	140	157
PROTEIN	2g	6g
FAT	5g	0.74g
SATURATED FAT	1g	0.12g
CHOLESTEROL	0mg	0mg
SODIUM	230mg	(you control the salt)
CARBOHYDRATES	22g	34g
FIBER	2g	6g
SUGAR	4g	0.39g

INGREDIENTS (WHEAT THINS): Whole-grain wheat flour, unbleached enriched flour (wheat flour, niacin, reduced iron, thiamine mononitrate [vitamin B_1], riboflavin [vitamin B_2], folic acid), soybean oil, sugar, cornstarch, malt syrup (from barley and corn), salt, invert sugar, leavening (calcium phosphate and/or baking soda), vegetable color (annatto extract, turmeric oleoresin). BHT added to packaging material to preserve freshness.

INGREDIENTS (WHEAT BERRIES): Wheat berries

SOURCES: NABISCO PRODUCT INFORMATION; THE USDA NATIONAL NUTRIENT DATABASE FOR STANDARD REFERENCE.

thing: A popular wheat cracker based on a percentage of ground wheat can be legally called a "100% whole-grain" food, and touted as such on the package. But the real deal has three times the fiber for starters, more protein, no sugar, and almost five times less fat, which is added during processing.

Similarly, compare flavored tortilla chips from a bag with the ones you can make in a few minutes. The differences are clear, especially when you consider these factors:

• The calorie count is almost the same, even though the serving size for homemade chips is twice as much by weight. And when you eat 2 ounces of real corn tortillas, you've actually eaten something.

Store-bought Chips vs. Homemade Chips

	DORITOS SALSA VERDE CHIPS (1 SERVING; ABOUT 12 CHIPS; 1 OUNCE)	VB6 TORTILLA CRISPS (PAGE 192; 1 SERVING; 2 WHOLE CORN TORTILLAS; ABOUT 2 OUNCES)
CALORIES	140	188
PROTEIN	2g	4g
FAT	7g	9g
SATURATED FAT	1g	1g
CHOLESTEROL	0mg	0mg
SODIUM	210mg	412mg
CARBOHYDRATES	19g	25g
FIBER	1g	4g
SUGARS	1g	2g

INGREDIENTS (DORITOS SALSA VERDE CHIPS): Whole corn, vegetable oil (corn, canola, soybean, and/or sunflower oil), maltodextrin (made from corn), salt, monosodium glutamate, dextrose, jalapeño pepper powder, tomato powder, paprika, onion, citric acid, modified cornstarch, natural and artificial flavors (including natural chicken flavor), spices, garlic, spice extractives, vinegar, corn syrup solids, artificial color (including Yellow 6 Lake, Red 40 Lake, Blue 1 Lake), parsley, lemon juice.

INGREDIENTS (VB6 TORTILLA CRISPS): Corn tortillas, tomato paste, olive oil, chili powder, salt, black pepper.

SOURCES: PEPSICO/FRITO-LAY PRODUCT INFORMATION; CALCULATED FROM THE USDA NATIONAL NUTRIENT DATABASE FOR STANDARD REFERENCE.

• No one actually eats a 1-ounce serving of Doritos, and if you eat 2 ounces, you'll double the calories, still want more, have eaten that much more of stuff like corn syrup, chicken flavor (what is that?), and artificial color, and you will have spent three bucks instead of twenty-five cents.

• With store-bought chips, fat is the overriding issue, and though the homemade version certainly isn't fat free, you're eating olive oil, which has both good flavor and a healthful nutritional profile.

• Once you know the nutritional and physiological differences between hyper-processed and whole foods, you have a choice. And if you want to lose or maintain your weight, you have to choose the right kinds of carbohydrates.

"GOOD" VERSUS "BAD" CARBS

For years carbohydrates have been referred to as either simple ("bad") or complex ("good"). The scientific distinction was that simple carbohydrates were sugars, like fructose (found in fruit), sucrose (table sugar, essentially, extracted from sugarcane or sugar beets), and dextrose and glucose (found in corn and grapes, among other things). Complex carbohydrates included foods that contained three or more sugars—pretty much everything else.

But this distinction is neither accurate nor helpful because not all so-called simple or complex carbohydrates are digested or metabolized—converted into energy—in the same way.

For example, the starch from white bread, technically a complex carb, is converted to blood sugar nearly as fast as pure glucose, a so-called simple carb. And the sugar in fruit (fructose, a simple carb) isn't converted quite as fast, or in the same way, as glucose. (Don't forget that the sugar in fruits comes along with fiber, water, and nutrients.)

So you can have "bad" complex carbs and "good" simple ones; and what that means is that we need to better judge what's bad and what's good. What follows is a summary of the current scientific thinking on this, and my conclusions about how (and which) carbs fit best into the VB6 diet.

Our bodies handle different types of carbohydrates differently based on their specific compositions of sugars, starches, and fiber. Studying these differences has become one of the most important and controversial areas of nutritional research. And since carbohydrates are an important and large part of our diets, we need to be aware of these differences not only in order to lose weight but to get the most nutrition from the foods we eat.

Let's start with sugar. Each of the different sugars described above as a "simple carbohydrate" is changed during digestion so that the body can use it efficiently. Most become glucose, the body's optimal fuel. Since glucose is water soluble, it's easily carried through the bloodstream, providing all of the body's cells—brain, muscles, organs—with the energy they need to function. (In fact "blood sugar" is glucose.) You don't have to be a scientist to understand that the easier a carbohydrate is to break down to glucose, the faster it will be digested and used as energy.

But you can have too much glucose—more than your body needs immediately—and that can cause problems. Because glucose can't be stored, a lengthy and complicated process eventually converts it to fat. Fat is an excellent storehouse for energy, so this makes perfect sense: Your body takes the energy it doesn't need and saves it to burn later, when it has a shortfall.

But most of us *never stop eating.* Once you already have "enough" energy to burn now, and adequate fat stored for the future, more sugar piles on more fat. To lose weight, you've got to not only eat fewer calories but less of the foods that are easiest to convert to glucose and stored fat. And the best way to do that is to minimize the amount of rapidly digestible excess glucose in your bloodstream.

This makes sense for another reason too: Besides being stored as fat, glucose (remember: blood sugar) stimulates the pancreas to secrete the hormone insulin. Insulin regulates blood sugar levels, making sure that the blood has enough glucose to provide energy for the body's cells. But it also helps determine how and when the body stores fat by triggering a complex chain reaction that's designed to regulate hunger and send out satiety signals. Put simply, less glucose (that is, less sugar and fewer hyper-processed carbs) equals less insulin production, and less of both results in less storage of fat.

When it works, as it does for most people most of the time, this chain reaction is an elegant and precise system. But the balance is delicate and for some people—those who either were born with problems producing and regulating insulin or who develop problems metabolizing glucose over a period of time—it can veer out of whack. The result is diabetes, either what's known as Type 1 (the kind you're born with or develop early in life) or Type 2. This second is the type that is raging in America, developing in both adults and children (even though it was until recently called "adult-onset diabetes"), often brought on by obesity that is in turn largely the result of consuming large quantities of processed carbohydrates.

It's likely you know how serious diabetes is, since it's likely you know someone with the disease: As of this writing, around 26 million Americans have Type 2 diabetes, and a whopping 79 million Americans have blood sugar issues that indicate pre-diabetes. (I was one of this latter group until I began the VB6 diet.)

INSULIN AND THE HUNGER HORMONES

Yet problems controlling blood sugar levels arise in almost all of us, whether we're diabetic or not. You have probably heard of hypoglycemia, a blood sugar condition that occurs when there is an imbalance between glucose and insulin levels. This might mean your glucose levels rise and plummet rapidly, or your glucose levels are too low and drop further, or your insulin levels are too high and rise higher, or a combination of these factors. If you consume carbohydrates that make your glucose and insulin levels spike (processed carbohydrates will do the trick), the sudden drop in blood sugar that ensues leaves you hungry, and sometimes dizzy and anxious, just one or two hours later. (Severe hypoglycemia can make you faint or even cause a seizure.)

How do you address hypoglycemia? Ironically, the easiest, most immediate way is to eat food with high levels of glucose, which is what you usually crave anyway. But if all you're eating is highly processed carbs with high glucose levels, this cycle of ups and downs never ends. As with many biological functions, maintaining consistent energy levels is a complicated system of checks and balances; but a change in diet can play a large role in controlling sudden hunger.

Hunger, of course, is your body's way of ensuring nourishment, but unfortunately this glucose-insulin spike-and-drop cycle can lead you to consume excess calories that your body has trouble processing. And if this cycle becomes chronic, you can develop insulin resistance, meaning the hormone can no longer efficiently regulate and store glucose, causing muscles and cells to "resist" the way insulin functions to control blood sugar.

One way to prevent and control high glucose and insulin levels and hypoglycemia (which can become chronic and very problematic) is to rely on carbohydrates that are digested and used by the body in a way that is similar to how a time-release drug works: slowly, consistently, and over longer periods of time. This means, for the most part, eating vegetables, legumes, and real whole grains.

Insulin is even more important than I've made it seem so far, because every molecule of energy that enters your body in the form of food is assigned to be either burned or stored; those are the only two options. As the regulator of the rate at which you burn and store calories for energy, insulin is the dominant factor in determining which of those options is chosen for every bite you eat. The more insulin present in your bloodstream, the more incoming energy will be converted to fat; less insulin means that more of that energy is burned immediately.

Meanwhile, fat cells produce and release a hormone called leptin, which also circulates in the blood. When leptin reaches high enough levels, it sends the message to your hypothalamus—a pearl-sized part of your brain—that you've stored enough energy. This is your body's signal to slow or stop eating. Leptin *usually* decreases your appetite, limiting your food intake, reducing your insulin levels and therefore the rate at which energy is converted to fat. In the long term, leptin helps manage your weight by informing your brain how much fat is available in your body.

Ghrelin, a hormone secreted in the stomach, is what makes you hungry in the first place. It kicks in whenever the body needs more glucose for energy, signaling the brain that it's time to eat. When your body is functioning well, the interactions among ghrelin, leptin, insulin, and the brain, pancreas, stomach, and your fat cells maintain an adequate but not superfluous supply of energy throughout the day— indeed, throughout your life.

But the interplay among insulin, ghrelin, and leptin is delicate, and since these three "hunger hormones" share communication pathways in the hypothalamus, an insulin malfunction has a cascading effect. For example, too much insulin can block leptin receptors in the brain, which in turn triggers erroneous signaling.

If your hypothalamus can't "see" your leptin, your brain continues to signal a lack of energy and will not only increase your appetite but reduce your activity level to conserve that energy. You can even become leptin resistant, which causes your hypothalamus to think that you are literally starving. When that happens, your body will do whatever it takes to get the glucose it needs and protect itself from starvation, and because of hormonal imbalances and resistance due to overconsumption, you may gain weight. Lots of weight—enough to become obese.

In recent years, researchers and pharmacological marketers realized that if they could develop a pill that increased our leptin signals, making us feel full faster, we would eat less and gain less weight, or even lose weight. Likewise a pill that reduced ghrelin levels should reduce hunger signals.

Both of these sound like miracle pills, and the company that successfully develops one is looking at a windfall. But as I said, this is an extremely complex mechanism that involves more than one isolated hormone, and we're far from fully understanding or being able to artificially manipulate our hunger and satiety signals. To date, the miracles remain forthcoming.

METABOLISM GONE WRONG

Of course, even being less hungry doesn't ensure that we'll eat nutritious food, and it's *what* we eat as well as how *much* we eat that represents the core problem. Which makes the solution far simpler than explaining the problem. You don't even need to fully understand this complex system to recognize that you ignore it at your own risk.

Obesity, or even being more than a little overweight, is a warning that the system isn't functioning properly, that you're not converting, burning, and storing the food you eat in an ideal fashion, and that you're at risk of developing a variety of diseases. There's a name for the downward spiral of risk factors that can lead to coronary disease, Type 2 diabetes, stroke, high blood pressure, and cholesterol issues: metabolic syndrome.

Obviously you want to avoid this, and doing so is almost as simple as reducing your intake of foods high in sugar and hyper-processed carbohydrates. Part of the trouble, however, is that many of the sugars in our diet (or foods that cause blood sugar levels to spike after eating) don't appear on labels as the word *sugar*.

Consider the now-infamous high fructose corn syrup (HFCS). This common ingredient has become so reviled that its producers tried to get its name legally changed to "corn sugar." (They failed.) Composed of 42 percent glucose and 55 to 58 percent fructose, HFCS is found in all sorts of processed foods in supermarkets and restaurants.

Glucose in the diet, as you now know, raises blood glucose levels to the point that sugar is converted to fat. And remember: Glucose also triggers insulin secretion, which should reduce your hunger as it helps your body process this sugar.

Fructose is a sugar, too, but it's handled differently: It's sent directly to the liver, where some of it is eventually converted to glucose. But because fructose isn't immediately converted to glucose, eating it doesn't stimulate insulin production right away, and therefore doesn't suppress hunger the same way glucose does. The fructose that isn't converted to glucose is, of course, metabolized into fat and stored.

So in a way, HFCS hits the body with a double whammy of fat potential: It doesn't suppress hunger and it may eventually be converted to fat. This is especially the case if you consume a lot of it. And it's even worse than that, because when HFCS is manufactured, the fructose itself is what you might call denatured: It's made easier to digest than "natural" fructose (the kind, for example, that you find in fruit), or even sucrose (the kind of sugar found in sugarcane and sugar beets), and so it wreaks even more havoc in your body. Furthermore, much HFCS is found in soda, and liquids do almost nothing to suppress hunger—so you "eat" HFCS without gaining any satiety. Did I say double whammy? Quadruple.

Our daily per capita consumption of *added* sugars—mostly HFCS and its relatives, the ones that dominate soda and many other hypersweet foods, and are hidden in countless other processed foods—is around 22 teaspoons, a whopping 355 calories' worth. So if you eliminate those sugars alone—and that's pretty much the sugars in junk food—you'll eliminate the equivalent of a pound's worth of calories (3,500) every ten days. Forever. Not a quick plan for weight loss, but in and of itself a smart one. And even if you replace some of those calories with real food, you'll be benefiting in two ways: a net calorie reduction, and the substitution of calories that are more likely to be beneficial or at least benign for those that can do you harm. This is another core principle of VB6.

THE SPECIAL CASE OF FRUIT

All this talk about fructose might give fruit a bad name because, as the name implies, fruit is where fructose occurs naturally. In fact, the more extreme anti-carbohydrate advocates do suggest limiting the amount of fruit you eat.

But fructose is problematic only in excessive quantities. And a piece of fruit contains relatively little fructose compared to sodas, packaged desserts, and other sweet snacks—exactly the stuff we eat too much of. One HFCS-sweetened 12-ounce can of cola, smaller than the 16- and 20-ounce bottles sold as single servings, contains roughly 40 grams of sugar, or about four times the amount in a large peach. And of those sugars, 22.45 grams of the cola's sugars come from fructose, while only 2.3 grams of the peach's sugars come from fructose. That's ten times more fructose in a can of Coke than in a peach, without any of the peach's benefits.

Since fruit also contains sucrose and glucose, the amount of naturally occurring fructose in any given type of fruit—even fruit with a relatively high percentage of fructose, like cherries or figs—remains quite small. Soda, like most processed snacks, is worth nothing nutritionally, whereas a peach contains only real ingredients, many of them—like fiber and micronutrients—inarguably good for you. Vital, even.

The bottom line is that not only are a few pieces of fruit a day *not* a problem but that fruit consumed *in place of soda* could single-handedly reduce obesity dramatically.

SLOW-BURNING STARCHES

Sugars aren't the only kind of carbohydrates that threaten our diet, so cutting out the obvious—sweetened "foods" like soda—is only the first step. We also have to discuss "starches," the so-called complex carbohydrates, which have been deceptively lumped together as "good" carbohydrates.

Starches are carbohydrates composed of chains of sugars, and like "simple" sugars, they're not all the same. Wheat, which we eat in many forms and which is a staple for many people around the world, is a fine example to explore. The wheat berry—the seed of the wheat plant—is a whole grain; only the chaff and stems have been removed. Each wheat berry has three layers: the outside (or bran), the middle layer (the bulk of the grain, called the endosperm), and the center (or germ). The bran and germ contain most of the nutrients, not only in wheat but in all grains.

Whole grains like the wheat berry are a terrific source of prolonged, sustained energy. When you cook and eat wheat berries (sadly, the least familiar wheat product), the body begins to convert most parts of the grain to glucose. But because the berry contains many other components—not just starch, but also protein and fiber—this happens slowly and provides a steady source of energy for several hours, *without* the sugar crashes associated with highly processed carbohydrates.

Hyper-process that wheat berry and everything changes. To make white flour, the bran and the germ are removed—the very parts that take the longest to digest—leaving the starchy endosperm and only a little of the kernel's fiber, protein, and fat. It's not surprising then that the starch in white flour is digested and converted rapidly; our bodies treat that starch more like sugars than like whole grains. The result is that hyper-processed grains can lead to the same glucose and insulin roller-coaster spikes and drops as sugar.

By now you've grasped the value of whole grains over hyper-processed grains. But despite what amounts to common knowledge we haven't succeeded in integrating whole grains into our diets; on average, we eat less than one serving of them a day. And it's not for lack of trying but for confusion. When the government (or any other entity) recommends that you eat "grains," you'd be perfectly sane in understanding that to mean "bread," or "pasta," or "rice." And when the recommendation becomes more specific and says eat "whole grains," you'd still not be faulted for thinking this meant so-called whole-grain or whole wheat bread.

This is a legal and a labeling problem, one exploited by food processors who market "whole grain" bread in a way that convinces people that by eating it they're consuming whole grains. But this is *absolutely* not the case: It's a very long way from a wheat berry to so-called whole-grain bread. In fact whole-grain bread has far more in common with white bread than it does with that wheat berry.

Commercial whole wheat flour at least contains the bran and germ, so it's a better choice over white flour. (Though it's not clear how much of the bran and germ are actually retained when industrial mills make "whole wheat" flour.) But the kernel is so broken down in the milling that it might be considered partially digested before you even start chewing it, making it easier for your body to convert it to glucose. And this efficiency isn't doing you any favors; it just means more sugar available all at once—sugar that might spike insulin and/or be converted to fat. Commercially processed whole wheat flour might be better than white flour, but it's still not a whole grain.

To ensure good health and increase the chances of weight loss, you've got to let your body—not big manufacturers—digest your food for you. The more you make your body work to convert what you eat to energy, the better the whole system works.

A WORD ABOUT FIBER

This brings us to fiber, a type of carbohydrate that the body cannot digest at all. Since it isn't converted to sugar to burn now or fat to store for later, it has no calories. How, you might ask (I did), can something that isn't digestible and doesn't provide energy be beneficial? (Come to think of it, fiber is a lot like water, and it may be helpful to think of it that way.) Read on.

Fiber is a coarse, strandlike material found in fruits, vegetables, whole grains, and legumes. Only whole fruits and vegetables have fiber; animal foods and fats contain no fiber. There are two kinds of fiber: soluble, which dissolves in water, and is found in most legumes, fruits, and oats; and insoluble, which does not dissolve in water and is a component of most grains, vegetables, and nuts. Soluble fiber helps lower cholesterol and glucose levels in the blood. Insoluble fiber creates bulk in the intestines and plays an important role in moving foods through your digestive tract. Most carbohydrates that contain fiber have both types. Besides improving digestion and helping prevent constipation, increased fiber in the diet can lower the risk for Type 2 diabetes and heart disease.

How much fiber is enough? The Department of Agriculture recommends at least 20 grams of total fiber a day for women and 30 grams for men; most Americans get less than 15 grams a day. And how much of each kind do you need? Doesn't matter: You need both. And you don't need to spend too much time thinking about this, because a diet with lots of fruits, vegetables, whole grains, and legumes—like VB6—provides enough fiber of both kinds. Period.

MEASURING HOW THE BODY BURNS CARBS

With all of these carbs offering varying levels of benefit and harm, researchers wanted to come up with a system that would quantify their effect on blood sugar. They came up with the glycemic index (GI) and glycemic load (GL)—measuring tools that offer partial solutions to the questions surrounding how carbohydrates are metabolized.

I bring up these two concepts because you're likely to run across them almost any time you read an intelligent examination of diet and nutrition, and they'll help you understand the origins of VB6 and why it's a sensible, sustainable way to eat, especially if you're trying to lose weight.

But VB6 is not *based* on either the GI or the GL, and you won't need to track any of these figures, ever. Still, like calorie density, the concepts are useful.

The glycemic index is a valuable way to demonstrate the difference between the effects of whole grains and refined (or "white") grains on your body's chemistry—to help differentiate "bad" carbs from "good." Foods with a high GI (over 70), like instant oatmeal and white rice, can dramatically increase blood sugar and insulin levels after meals, especially when eaten frequently.

Frequency is key: Foods with a high GI will always raise glucose and insulin levels, but if you eat them only once in a while, your body should be able to cope with these spikes. If, on the other hand, you eat them all the time, insulin will eventually struggle with the onslaught of glucose and become less capable of regulating it; this will in turn disrupt the way your cells, muscles, and organs absorb and use energy. The result can be insulin resistance, weight gain, and even diabetes.

Foods with a low GI (less than 55; between 55 and 70 is "moderate"), like legumes and most vegetables and fruits, don't spike blood sugar levels as quickly, and provide that desirable slow and consistent energy source without sudden sugar crashes. The index demonstrates that labeling carbs either "simple" or "complex" is not a valid distinction. (The whole thing would be much easier to understand if it were!) But since only one point separates "low" from "medium" and "medium" from "high," the categories are imprecise at best, so it's better to list them by their numeric values.

The Glycemic Index for Select Foods

FOOD ITEM	GLYCEMIC INDEX VALUE	FOOD	GLYCEMIC INDEX VALUE
Olive oil	These foods, when eaten alone, are not likely to induce a significant rise in blood glucose.	Whole wheat spaghetti	37 to 45
Vegetable oil (grapeseed oil)		Apples (without skin)	38
Chicken breast		Strawberries	40
Fillet of fish (bluefish, raw)		Apple juice	40
Bacon (cooked)		Twix	44
Parmesan cheese		White flour spaghetti (cooked)	41 to 58
Egg (hard-boiled)		Bulgur (cooked)	46
Tofu	15	Quinoa (uncooked)	53
Spinach	15	Corn	60
Tomatoes	15	Sweet potatoes (cooked)	61
Celery	15	Brown rice (cooked)	62
Iceberg lettuce	15	Coca-Cola (12 ounces)	63
Broccoli	15	Beets	64
Grapefruit	25	Special K cereal	69
Cashews	25	White rice	69
Dried apples	29	White flour	70
Black beans (cooked)	30	Commercial whole wheat bread	71
Lentils (cooked)	30	White bread	73
Milk (1% fat)	32	Pretzels	83
Carrots	35	Gatorade	89
Quinoa (cooked)	35	Regular potatoes (cooked)	98
Chickpeas (cooked)	36		

SOURCES: HARVARD MEDICAL SCHOOL, HARVARD HEALTH, "GLYCEMIC INDEX AND GLYCEMIC LOAD FOR 100+ FOODS"; SOUTH BEACH DIET PLAN; GLYCEMICINDEX.COM; THE MONTIGNAC METHOD DATABASE OF GLYCEMIC INDICES. (ONE OF THE DOWNFALLS OF GI CALCULATIONS IS THAT THEY ARE BASED ON AVERAGE LEVELS OF BLOOD SUGAR MEASURED AFTER PEOPLE EAT CERTAIN FOODS, SO THE VALUES FROM DIFFERENT SOURCES CAN VARY.)

You see all this when you look at the list of GIs for a variety of foods on the opposite page. These are the same foods selected to demonstrate calorie density on page 33.

WHERE THE GI FALLS SHORT

As you can see, highly processed carbohydrates tend to make for foods with a higher GI. The trouble is that a lot of whole grains fall into that moderately high territory, right up there with their refined counterparts, and that might discourage people from eating these important foods. Also, blindly following the chart would encourage you to consider a Twix bar (for example) a "good" food—because it's a low-GI food.

And this is precisely where the GI runs into problems. The unrefined (whole-grain) counterparts of white flour and white rice contain more fiber and protein and thus are, as I mentioned earlier, digested more slowly. So not only are whole grains more nutritious than highly processed grains, but studies continue to demonstrate that consuming *real* whole grains in place of hyper-processed ones can reduce the risk of many diseases and conditions: Type 2 diabetes and insulin sensitivity, strokes, heart disease, colorectal cancer, and high blood pressure. Real whole grains also aid in weight management and promote overall health.

The takeaway from all this is that GI is valuable but should not be taken as gospel and cannot be taken by itself. Some desirable foods— watermelon (72), bananas (62), and brown rice (60), for example—have a medium or even a high glycemic index, while many junk foods have a low or medium glycemic index. Strawberries and a Snickers bar have essentially the same glycemic index (40 and 41), yet the candy has practically no nutrients while a strawberry is packed with vitamins and fiber. To muddy the waters even further, note that Gatorade— essentially sugar water—has a high GI because of its sugar, but a low caloric density because it's mostly water.

The shortcomings of the GI led to the development of the glycemic load (GL), which calculates the amount of carbohydrates in food along with the impact of those carbohydrates on blood sugar levels. (To get at this number—not that you'd ever do it—you multiply the glycemic index of a food by the amount of carbohydrate it contains, and divide that number by 100. The final number should fall between from 0 and 30.)

A Candy Bar vs. Fruit		
	TWIX (2 COOKIES)	STRAWBERRIES (1 CUP SLICED)
CALORIES	250	53
FAT	12g	0.5g
SATURATED FAT	9g	0g
CARBOHYDRATES	33g	12.75g
SUGARS	24g	8.12g
FIBER	1g	3.3g
PROTEIN	2g	1g

SOURCE: MARS/TWIX PRODUCT INFORMATION; USDA NATIONAL NUTRIENT DATABASE FOR STANDARD REFERENCE.

This revised glycemic calculation works, sort of, as you'll see if we revisit the strawberry (4 calories per strawberry, so 40 calories for a serving of 10 strawberries) and the Twix bar (250 calories). The strawberry has a low glycemic load of 3, while the candy has a medium to high glycemic load of 18. This disparity may by now seem not only logical but obvious and reassuring. Thus, GL is a better indicator than the GI. But it, too, has drawbacks.

For one thing, you need to know a food's glycemic index to calculate its glycemic load. So if the GI is unreliable to begin with, the GL also will be flawed. To further muddle matters, the terms glycemic index and glycemic load are often used interchangeably because they both calculate the rise in blood sugar.

There's another big problem with these numbers: Neither provides any measurement for foods that don't contain carbohydrates. Indeed, the underpinning of this approach is that everything other than carbohydrates—like fats and animal proteins—is unlimited; you can eat as much of these foods as you like. The famous Atkins and other early no- or low-carb diets are all based on this premise.

This is unjustifiable, for those reasons discussed earlier. Though many people lose weight on low-carb diets, you'll gain weight as soon as you reintroduce the carbs into your diet. And most people who go on low-carb diets eventually fall back on bad habits, reverting to eating processed carbs instead of developing a new way of eating that is supported by carbohydrates that are actually beneficial. Furthermore, eating unlimited amounts of animal products can have other negative effects on the body (like, oh, heart disease), not to mention the enormous negative environmental impact.

The bottom line on GI and GL is that either can serve as a useful reference, but it's far easier to just choose minimally processed foods and whole foods—even fruits—over junk. That's why VB6 is informed by these tools (and calorie density), but doesn't rely wholly on any of them. And VB6 parts ways with the glycemic measurements on the value of carbohydrates, where it more closely draws from the principles of calorie density. Finally, it takes a very different direction when it comes to the second macronutrient found in food: fat.

THE IMPORTANCE OF FATS

Fat is another macronutrient that for decades has been subject to fluctuating, conflicting, often downright wrong theories, though perhaps it's slightly less confounding than carbs. And fortunately, current research has forced a dramatic change to how scientists view the role fat plays in health and weight loss, and the important relationship between fat and carbohydrates.

Fat, of course, is the greasy stuff found in all animals and almost all plants. Even the least calorie-dense foods, like spinach or blueberries, contain a teeny bit of fat, since all living things need it to function. By happy coincidence, fat also makes nearly everything taste better.

For years scientists maintained that fat had no taste because our taste buds, they said, recognize only sweet, salty, bitter, sour, and most recently, umami. But recent studies suggest that our tongues apparently can also discern fat and our taste buds have an affinity for its taste. So when fat is removed from naturally fatty foods—like, say, milk and cookies—you can easily recognize the difference; and more often than not, the low-fat version doesn't make the taste-bud cut. You've noticed, no doubt, that low-fat or fat-free foods are not as flavorful as their full-fat counterparts; nor do they feel as satisfying in the mouth, not to mention the stomach.

One thing about fat is inarguable: Of all the macronutrients, it's the most calorie-dense, clocking in at 9 calories per gram. That's not the whole story, though. The big questions, the ones that concern so many of us, are these: How is fat processed and stored? What's the difference between fat in the diet and fat in the body? After fat is stored, how do we burn it? (That is, once we put it on, how do we take it off?) Because as essential as fat is—and it's especially important for maintaining and developing the brain, which is about 60 percent fat—too much of it stored in the body can be harmful.

Scientists estimate that fat should constitute 3 to 5 percent of a man's body weight; for women, it's 12 to 15 percent. This essential fat is what the body needs to build cells, protect the nerves and organs (especially kidneys, liver, heart, and intestines), help hormones work properly, store many vitamins, insulate your insides, keep your skin and hair healthy, and—somewhat ironically—keep your appetite in check. Once these activities are taken care of, the remaining fat is stored in fat cells and in the liver, in the event that it's needed for energy at a later time.

Fat cells have roles other than storing energy, too. For one thing, you need fat to absorb and process many micronutrients, including vitamins. Depending on their molecular structure, these micronutrients are either fat- or water-soluble, meaning they require the presence of one or the other to become usable. Water-soluble nutrients and vitamins—like B complex vitamins and vitamin C—get dissolved in water and are eliminated in urine, so we need to replenish these daily.

When you ingest fat-soluble micronutrients, however—like vitamins A, D, K, and E—fat carries them through the bloodstream and makes them available to the cells that need them. The body uses some right away, storing the rest for later use in fatty tissues and the liver. For this reason, a well-nourished person doesn't need to consume fat-soluble nutrients daily. (In fact, these vitamins can be toxic when consumed in excess, though this is not something most people need to worry about.) Fat also carries fat-soluble hormones, like steroid hormones, thyroid hormones, and the sex hormones estrogen and testosterone. Minerals like calcium and magnesium also need fat to be absorbed and transported through the body.

So you *need* fat: It's crucial for fueling and nourishing all of the cells in your body (fat also helps regulate what goes in and out of our cells). You just don't need excess fat.

HOW FAT IS METABOLIZED

Nutrients are rarely if ever eaten in isolation, and the interplay among carbohydrates, protein, and fat affects how fat behaves in the body. In fact, the "hunger hormones"—insulin, leptin, and ghrelin—are interconnected (see page 40) and deal with the energy from fat and carbohydrates simultaneously.

Let's start by taking a look at what happens when you eat fat. You'll remember that we store unused fuel in the form of fat, to be reconverted to energy if and when we need it, but that one of our problems is that most of us rarely if ever go truly hungry and are forced to burn fat. Yet shrinking our swollen fat cells is key to losing weight.

Much as carbs are converted during digestion into glucose, fats are broken down into fatty acids, a form the body can use. These fatty acids are stored in fat cells, receptacles throughout the body that are designed for this specific purpose. The fat cells expand as fatty acids are deposited, so you can actually see excess calories set aside for future use.

Once any immediately "unneeded" fat is deposited in fat cells, it's all the same sort of raw energy; it doesn't matter if it started its life as fatty acids or as glucose from carbohydrates. What does matter is that as long as there is glucose circulating in the bloodstream, that's what the body will use for energy; the fat will sit there until called to action, which may be never. If at some point in the future, the glucose levels digested from eating carbohydrates drop enough in the bloodstream, insulin levels will also go down, and this drop in insulin means that fat cells will finally be called upon to release their reserved fuel. Only then—as the fat cells shrink—will the stored fat begin to melt away.

FAT IN OUR DIET

We know, then, that fat is essential, and that accumulating too much fat (or eating the wrong *kind* of fat; we'll get to that)—is not a good thing. But the science about this is in constant flux, and evolving quickly.

In the 1980s and early '90s, low-fat diets were all the rage, not just to lose weight but (in theory) to reduce the risk of heart disease. As a result, Americans eat far less fat than we did fifty years ago. In the '60s, we got 45 percent of our calories from fat; now we get a little more than 30 percent of calories from fat.

But something has gone wrong: More than 35 percent of American adults are now obese; in the '60s, when we ate much more fat, only 13 percent of us were obese. The rate of obesity has more than doubled in only fifty years.

What happened? As fat became demonized and its consumption plummeted, the consumption of carbohydrates skyrocketed: Our consumption of hyper-processed grains and sweeteners has gone up more than 40 percent over this same period of time.

Remember that we now get more than 50 percent of our calories from carbohydrates, and many of those are damaging sugars and hyper-processed grains. In the name of a "healthy, low-fat diet" we've devoured a category of carbohydrates that didn't even exist until quite recently; we've experimented on ourselves with an unprecedented, novel, and unique diet of unnatural foods, largely in the name of reducing our fat intake. (That's the SAD, the Standard American Diet, at work again.)

It's been a terrible swap. Current research increasingly indicates that drastically reducing your intake of fat is not necessarily the best way to lose weight, especially not if you're exchanging fat for a lot of carbohydrates with a high glycemic index. If you reduce fat and *don't* eat more of other foods, you will, of course, lose weight. But that isn't what most people have done.

In fact, the most recent evidence shows that high amounts of fat in a diet—in the range of 40 to 50 percent—aren't necessarily linked to weight gain and disease. However, the *type* of fat you eat matters a lot. So although we're eating less fat, the combination of more hyper-processed carbohydrates and the wrong fats is what's killing us.

Simply put: The fats you get from animal products, the fats you get from eating junk food (even "vegetable-based" junk food like chips), are worse for you than those found in nuts or olives or avocados—or the fats found in vegetables and grains. As with carbohydrates, the body doesn't treat all fats the same way. (More about that later.) For now, no discussion of fat can go far without addressing cholesterol, a waxy, fat-like substance found in animal foods.

UNDERSTANDING CHOLESTEROL

Cholesterol has gotten a bad reputation, but it's a crucial building block for cell membranes and a variety of the hormones we need for normal functioning. Our bodies make about 75 percent of the cholesterol that we need, mostly in the liver; we get the rest from food.

Like fat, cholesterol is essential to human life. But unlike carbohydrates and most proteins, neither fat nor cholesterol is water soluble, so a system is needed to make them bio-available. And the system that's evolved in humans is one in which the body coats them with protein, creating tiny particles called lipoproteins, which can then be transported via the bloodstream. There are many lipoproteins, but we focus on three types: low-density lipoproteins (LDL), high-density lipoproteins (HDL), and triglycerides.

Everyone who's paid attention to his or her blood work is familiar with these terms, but not everyone knows what they mean. LDL and HDL carry cholesterol throughout the body via the bloodstream. They work like this: LDL extracts fat and cholesterol from the liver as needed and carries them—via the bloodstream—to the body's cells. When too much LDL cholesterol remains in the bloodstream, these particles can form deposits called plaque on the inside walls of arteries, clogging them to varying degrees. This restriction of blood flow exacerbates high blood pressure, and the reverse is also true: High blood pressure can increase the likelihood of developing plaque. Either way, the condition can lead to a heart attack, stroke, or other cardiovascular complications. For this reason, LDL cholesterol is often called "bad" cholesterol.

On the other hand, HDL is called "good" cholesterol because it hunts down LDL cholesterol, whether it's in the bloodstream or stuck to the arteries' walls; it removes it and takes it back to the liver, where it can be reprocessed. In this way, HDL protects the body from the negative effects of LDL cholesterol—or tries to. This is why many people believe that total cholesterol—HDL plus LDL—is not as important a number as the ratio of good cholesterol to bad.

Fat triglycerides are mostly metabolized as fatty acids and glycerol, substances that the blood can easily transport—along with whatever fat-soluble nutrients come along for the ride—to all the cells that need them. (Fatty acids are stored in fat cells and glycerol is predominantly stored in the liver.) So even though triglycerides are important, too much of them is dangerous, and they're a good indicator of how effective your body is at processing fats and carbohydrates: Elevated levels of triglycerides can indicate risk for metabolic syndrome, insulin resistance, and Type 2 diabetes or other obesity-related diseases.

TYPES OF FAT

The food you eat contains different types of fat that behave differently during digestion and metabolism. As with carbohydrates, it's tempting to talk about them in terms of "good" and "bad"—or, rather, good, not good, and awful. But of course it's more complicated than that.

A little chemistry is in order here. Fat molecules are chains of carbon and hydrogen with oxygen tagged on at one end. How these strings of elements are put together determines how they react with other compounds in your body, and whether they're characterized as unsaturated, saturated, or hydrogenated fats. Most fats are a combination of all three (there are subcategories, too, as you'll see in a bit), but they are largely grouped by whatever type of fat is dominant.

Unsaturated fats are mostly found in foods derived from plants, and we see them in the oils made from vegetables, nuts, and seeds; they're easy to distinguish because they're all liquid at room temperature. Unsaturated fats fall into two groups: monounsaturated and polyunsaturated. Olives and olive oil, avocados, peanuts, almonds, hazelnuts and their oils, sesame and pumpkin seeds and the oil that comes from them, and canola oil all contain high proportions of monounsaturated fat.

Polyunsaturated fats are most commonly found in sunflower, corn, soybean, and flaxseed oils, and also in walnuts and fish, which is the primary nonplant source of unsaturated fat. Canola oil is also a good source of polyunsaturated fat.

Polyunsaturated fats are good sources of omega-3 and omega-6 essential fatty acids, called "essential" because your body needs them but can't produce them, so you've got to get them from food. Omega-6 fatty acids are easy to get (and most of us are currently getting too many of them); they're in virtually all unsaturated fats, especially vegetable and seed oils. Omega-3s are tougher to come by, especially in plant foods, but they're extremely valuable because they help reduce inflammation and lower the levels of LDL cholesterol and triglycerides in the bloodstream. Good food sources for omega-3 fatty acids are oily fish like salmon, mackerel, and sardines as well as walnuts and flax seeds.

Until recently, monounsaturated fats were considered the best types of fat to consume, and they are still recognized as crucial for good health. But polyunsaturated fats are increasingly seen as playing an important role in improving blood cholesterol levels and blood pressure; controlling inflammation; stabilizing heart rhythms; and protecting against all kinds of diseases: cancers, cardiovascular diseases, coronary heart disease—you name it. For these reasons, it makes sense to eat a balance of unsaturated fats.

It also makes sense to substitute both mono- and polyunsaturated fats for saturated fats as often as possible. Saturated fats, solid at room temperature, are found in animal products like meat, cheese, milk, cream, butter, and eggs; they're also found in some tropical oils like coconut or palm oil. It almost goes without saying that by reducing the amount of animal products in your diet, VB6 reduces your consumption of saturated fats.

THE DANGER OF TRANS FAT

There's a fourth category of fat that with any luck will soon become a nonissue, because banning it entirely would be a major step forward in public health. These are the so-called trans fats (technically called trans fatty acids), present in small quantities in dairy, meat, and other animal foods (they're created in the stomach of cows and other animals). The ones that most concern us, however, are man-made, like solid shortening—the kind used for frying or pie dough—or margarine. These are partially hydrogenated vegetable oils, and they are, quite simply, worse than useless; they're harmful.

The hydrogenation process makes liquid oil solid at room temperature, opaque, more stable, and less likely to go rancid. It makes liquid oil behave more like lard or butter, enhancing the flakiness of crackers and other baked or fried foods while increasing their shelf life. In restaurants, trans fats are often used for deep-frying because the partially hydrogenated oil can withstand being heated multiple times without altering its chemical composition. Generally, trans fats are cheap and reliable, so ideal for industrial processors of food.

Butter is more expensive and temperamental, and lard has been out of favor because it's high in saturated fat. But you're probably better off with butter or lard. Trans fatty acids have been shown to spike levels of LDL (bad) cholesterol in the blood and lower HDL (good) cholesterol, a combination that has been linked with an increased risk of heart disease and a host of other complications. Since labeling for trans fats is now required on packaged food (but not, as of this writing, on restaurant menus), they've become far less common than they were a decade ago. But they're still around, and are best avoided entirely.

CARBOHYDRATES AND CHOLESTEROL

As you probably know, saturated fat, the subject of intense research for decades, was first deemed harmful because it was thought to raise blood cholesterol, at least in some people. And maybe it does.

But it now appears that that same excessive intake of hyper-processed carbohydrates that increases the chance of insulin resistance also triggers the liver to manufacture cholesterol, specifically the undesirable LDL cholesterol. And substituting carbohydrates for fats reduces the amount of (good) HDL cholesterol and therefore increases the risk of heart disease. Once again, carbohydrates and fat are closely linked; it's difficult to address one without the other.

When the Atkins and like diets heavily reliant on animal protein, and therefore saturated fat, claimed that they did not cause the other health complications thought to be brought about by saturated fat but were indeed beneficial because they reduced the risk of diabetes and obesity, eager dieters latched on to them. And certainly many people on Atkins-like diets did lose weight—at least in the short term—without raising their cholesterol levels. But besides being difficult to stick to, Atkins-like diets have been associated with a variety of health problems, beginning with the inflammation thought to be at the root of heart disease. And as it turns out, eating unsaturated fats in lieu of saturated fats has been proven to lower (bad) LDL cholesterol and increase (good) HDL cholesterol, which helps lower the risk of metabolic syndrome, especially heart disease, insulin resistance, and thus Type 2 diabetes.

Fat is essential for survival, so avoiding it is not a wise move from either the weight-loss or general health perspective. And current research is nearly unanimous in agreeing that it's more important for good health to minimize the refined carbohydrates in your diet for all the reasons covered earlier. But instead of replacing carbohydrates with animal protein and saturated fat, it's best to turn to a balanced diet with a combination of healthier fats—like those found in olive and seed oils, nuts, avocados, and oily fish—and minimally processed plants and whole grains.

Do that, and the majority of your fat will come from plants in the form of unsaturated fat, and few of your carbs will be hyper-processed— exactly what will naturally happen on a VB6 diet. With its more holistic and less obsessive approach to eating, with its minimized animal food consumption, VB6 allows you to eat without considering every bite and still manages to alter the balance of your fat intake so that you'll be eating a wide variety of the right kind of fats *and* carbs. (On top of that, cutting out hyper-processed food will eliminate the dreaded trans fats, which are by far the worst for you.)

Overall, VB6 focuses on plant-based fats that enhance the flavor and nutrition of all those vegetables, beans, and whole grains you'll be eating. And throughout the day, these will become your primary sources of protein.

THE PROTEIN MYTH

Like carbohydrates and fats, protein is found in almost every part of your body. It's used for maintenance and repair, particularly in muscles, bones, skin, and hair, but also in blood and organ tissue. It's also needed to keep many chemical reactions running smoothly, including the all-important part of your blood that carries oxygen around. But unlike carbohydrates and fats, you don't consume whole protein directly and it isn't stored in the body in any form.

Instead the body manufactures protein—more than 10,000 different types—by stringing together amino acids. Your body manufactures some amino acids, but around twenty are called "essential" because your body cannot produce them; you must get these from food. So you've got to eat protein almost daily in order to live. That's undeniable.

That doesn't mean you need as much as most Americans get, and I call this section "The Protein Myth" because for decades we've been encouraged to eat way more protein than we need, and we're eating more every year. According to the Census Bureau, since 1980 we've increased our annual per capita consumption of red meat, poultry, fish, and seafood by 11 pounds. (The type has shifted a little, however, away from red meat and toward poultry.) We consume a couple of dozen fewer eggs per year since then, but we eat a whopping 64 more pounds of dairy in the form of milk, cheese, yogurt, ice cream, and so on.

As a result, each American eats on average almost 800 pounds of protein-heavy animal products a year, more than 2 pounds every day, or as much as 6 ounces (more than 160g) of pure protein. And that provides way more protein than we need, perhaps twice or even three times as much.

So protein is another nutrient that's been misunderstood, and though the problem is perhaps not as intractable, the results can be equally dangerous. But like all questions of nutrition, that of how much protein we need each day to keep the machine running well is not an easy one.

PLANTS HAVE PROTEIN, TOO

The usual recommendation is for a little less than a gram of protein for every kilogram of body weight. That works out to 58 or so grams a day for a 160-pound adult. (To put this in perspective, there's about 1 ounce [28 grams] of protein in 5 ounces of chicken breast or lean beef.)

But according to the Harvard School of Public Health, adults typically get 15 percent of their daily calories from protein; if you're eating

2,000 calories a day, that's about 75 grams of protein, well over what you need. And since most people eat way more than 2,000 calories a day, many of us get something like twice the amount of protein we need, even by the already liberal gram per kilo estimate. Some experts argue that the amount of protein we eat is dangerously high, enough to cause a mineral imbalance or even be toxic. I'm not convinced that's the case, but I *am* convinced that most of us could thrive on about half the protein we're taking in now.

The overage is no surprise. For years the USDA dietary guidelines, inexpensive fast food, and a string of popular diet books have all encouraged us to get our protein by chowing down on burgers, chicken, eggs, and double-cheese pizza, all washed down with glasses of milk and followed by ice cream. Animal products are promoted as *the* way to get protein. (It's not exactly a criminal conspiracy, but it is a well-coordinated marketing effort spurred by enormous profits.) And, indeed, those are high-protein foods, and they're full of vitamins. And hormones, antibiotics, saturated fat, and, in their fast- or convenience-food form, hyper-processed carbohydrates. But not only can you get those vitamins and minerals from plants, you can get protein too—along with phytonutrients not found in meat.

In fact, plants can provide comparable nutrition to animal protein, and without the downsides; many plants have *more* protein per calorie than meat. Let's highlight some numbers from the chart on page 62: A cheeseburger contains about 0.04 grams of protein per calorie, and raw spinach has about 0.12 grams of protein per calorie—three times as much. Of course, since spinach is so low in calories you'd need to eat much more to get a comparable amount of protein, but that's easily done—a pound of spinach cooks down to next to nothing.

And in that pound of spinach, you'll find 100 calories—and therefore 13 grams of protein—10 grams of fiber, 17 grams of carbohydrates, 2 grams of fat, 0 grams of saturated fat, and a spectrum of vitamins and nutrients.

The cheeseburger, in comparison, which weighs 119g, contains over 300 calories—13 grams of protein—1.3 grams of fiber, 33.09 grams of carbohydrates, 7.4 grams of sugar (there's none in the spinach), 14 grams of fat, and 5.2 grams of saturated fat.

How Much Protein Is in That?

	CHEESE-BURGER	CHICKEN BREAST	PINTO BEANS	TOFU	BROCCOLI	RAW SPINACH
Protein per gram	0.13	0.16	0.09	0.08	0.02	0.03
Protein per calorie	0.04	0.23	0.06	0.11	0.07	0.12

SOURCE: USDA NATIONAL NUTRIENT DATABASE FOR STANDARD REFERENCE.

So you can get adequate protein from high-quality food or an over-adequate amount from low-quality food. VB6 is about making that first choice as often as possible; and when you do, it can have a huge and positive impact on your health.

What about the essential amino acids that you can get only from meat? Turns out this well-known "fact" isn't true: If you're eating a well-balanced diet of any sort—including a vegan diet—you'll get all the essential amino acids you need. Nor do you need to cover all the bases during any given meal; eating a variety of foods throughout the day will do the trick.

And there are benefits to substituting plant for animal protein. This is especially true of the protein found in beans; their high levels of fiber can lower cholesterol and blood pressure and reduce the risk of diabetes, and even treat the disease where it already exists. But although there's always been anecdotal evidence that vegans and even vegetarians tend to be leaner than meat-eaters, recently a reputable study tracked people over time and found that subjects gained weight—typically about 30 pounds—when their diets went from plant-based to meat-based; their health deteriorated as well. It's always difficult to prove causation, but even after controlling for other factors, vegans and dairy-and-egg–eating vegetarians had 50 percent less Type 2 diabetes.

This doesn't address protein directly, of course, but it does seem safe to say that you don't *need* animal products—or much of them—for good health. Even an all-vegan diet provides you with all the high-quality protein you need, and a diet that contains any animal products at all—even a couple of ounces a day—is really just added insurance. And that's just what VB6 gives you.

THE KEY TO FEELING FULL

No diet will work if you're "starving." You have to feel satisfied—satiated—both physiologically and psychologically. And eating a well-balanced diet of real food will do that for you while helping reduce cravings, especially for junk.

Short-term diets are easy. "I'm going to cut out all carbs for two weeks" sounds doable to anyone. Yet feeling deprived (or worse, hungry) while dieting—which you most certainly will if you cut out carbs—simply isn't sustainable in the long run: Neither your body nor your mind can endure it.

Which is why these diets fail. We covered how your body copes with a prolonged state of hunger by storing more energy, slowing your metabolism in an attempt to gain weight. Just as important, though, are the psychological effects of deprivation. You may feel frustrated, fatigued, anxious, maybe even depressed with a restrictive diet.

THE CONCEPT OF SATIETY

There's a difference between being full and being satisfied. You may indeed feel full—stuffed—after a breakfast of a poofy bagel with a couple of ounces of cream cheese; it is, after all, 370 calories. But since it's high in refined carbs, low in fiber, and lacks many of the nutrients your body needs for efficient fuel, the bulk of its calories come from starches that will immediately be broken down into sugar and trigger an insulin spike, guaranteeing that you'll be hungry again within a couple of hours.

Actual satiety means feeling comfortably satisfied for a while without sugar crashes. And one key to VB6 is to rely on foods that not only fill you up but also keep you satisfied. Protein and fat—whether from animals or plants—are digested more slowly and are therefore most satisfying; minimally processed carbs (vegetables, whole grains, even fruits) come next. Not surprisingly, hyper-processed carbohydrates, with their quick-burning sugars, are generally the least satiating foods you can eat.

Remember that not all carbohydrates are equal. Those that are high in fiber, which isn't processed into fuel but pretty much passes through your digestive system, are especially satisfying for their sheer bulk. It may not be a pleasant image, but because fiber has no calories, absorbs water, and isn't itself absorbed, it's a bit like eating a sponge that sits there taking up room—and then leaves. Because fiber is processed slowly, foods containing it have staying power, keeping you full for long stretches. This is why refined carbohydrates are the least filling of all foods, and why a bowl of real oatmeal keeps you full longer than a bagel.

Fibrous carbohydrates also require more chewing time than other foods, which means more eating satisfaction. Long chewing slows down the rate at which you swallow, giving your stomach some time to send its "I'm full" signals, which in turn can help minimize your intake. Think about the satisfaction of eating an apple versus drinking a glass of apple juice; that's about fiber. (The apple has 4.4 grams; a cup of juice 0.5 grams; the juice, by the way, also contains more sugar.)

I can't say this enough ways: Whole foods are more nutritious, provide better fuel, and are more filling than their processed counterparts. It's the naturally occurring fiber of grains, fruits, and vegetables that makes them satisfying.

There's no question that animal products are filling: The combination of fat and protein does the trick. But high-protein plants combined with high-quality oils and whole grains are equally satisfying, without the downside of saturated fat or the many horrors of industrial animal production.

Stick to beans, whole grains, and vegetables cooked with olive or good vegetable oil, and you have the basis for meals and snacks that satisfy both your physical and your mental cravings, since you'll be sitting in front of an attractive, fragrant, flavorful, and substantial plate of food. For your sugar cravings, fruit—and plenty of it.

THE TWO V'S

As we all know—all too well—the sheer volume of food is part of what satisfies us, especially psychologically: The amount you eat is essential to feeling full, regardless of the actual food item or calorie density of the food; and eating abundantly is a hardwired pleasure—a universal craving. So eating large quantities of foods with low calorie density—this means fruits and vegetables, which usually feature a great deal of volume with relatively few calories—can help make small portions of protein and fat more satisfying. (This is why vegetable-based soups or salads are a boon for anyone trying to lose weight, and the perfect way to start a meal, for all of these reasons.) It also allows you to eat pretty much as often and as much as you feel is necessary (within reason, of course), as long as you limit the meat and the junk. Do that, and you're not likely to gain weight. In fact, you'll probably lose it.

Successful weight loss is a game not only of volume but of variety. Your mind must register that what's on your plate is going to be satisfying, but if you eat too much of the same thing, a sort of defense mechanism called sensory-specific satiety kicks in and makes you full, preventing you from overloading on any one nutrient. As you eat the same food, the pleasure you derive from it declines with every bite. Basically, your body is causing you to get sick of it, signaling that you should eat a balanced and varied diet, increasing your chances of getting all the nutrients you need for good functioning from different foods.

That's why not many people actually eat ten chocolate chip cookies or one 24-ounce Porterhouse in one sitting; after a few bites our bodies begin to reject those high concentrations of identical nutrients. (Of course, plenty of people overrule these sensations, eating a couple of dozen cookies or finishing that steak. If, however, leptin is doing its job, they'll feel full bordering on sick. When leptin or insulin are out of whack, though, chronic overeating can result.)

You can use sensory-specific satiety to your advantage, because your body will feel full after eating a large quantity of *anything*, regardless of its calorie density. When you eat a large portion of low-calorie-dense food—again, we're talking about fruits and vegetables—that sensory-specific satiety will still kick in, but you've eaten fewer calories.

How is it that we always have room for dessert? Because we're capable of overriding our leptin signals, especially when we're tempted by food's pleasurable (or addictive) properties. Also, because dessert is a "new" food that adds variety to the end of the meal, sensory-specific satiety is weakened. But the sick feeling of eating too much—that physical malaise that results from leptin screaming for you to stop—will probably still be there.

VB6 METABOLISM

Let's see what all of this theory looks like in practice when it comes to a meal: You might start by eating some vegetable soup—get some water and fiber in that stomach and start to signal fullness. (Studies show that starting a meal with salad or with soup actually helps you eat less of the main course.) Next would come calorie-dense foods—say, a brown rice pilaf cooked with beans or tofu—accompanied by a mound of spinach sautéed in olive oil or sliced tomatoes, or both; since they both have low calorie densities, it doesn't matter much.

This is, in fact, a large meal, and your mind will register that, while the variety will leave you full, nourished, and satisfied with the array of textures and flavors, the calorie intake will be quite moderate. And you'll stay full for hours, thanks to the balance of high protein, water, fiber, slow-burning whole grains, and unsaturated fats, while avoiding sugar crashes from processed carbohydrates. A non-vegan, post-6 P.M. meal would look much the same, but perhaps with a bit of meat in it.

In short, VB6 does not mean eating less (in fact, your volume of food may increase) but rather shifting the balance of foods you eat to lower the overall calorie density of the meal.

It concerns some people that VB6 generally makes dinner the largest meal. As everyone knows, nighttime is a pitfall of second helpings, salty snacks, and sweet desserts, and continuing to eat after dinner can pack on pounds fast. So if you can head off this late-night eating cycle, you'll end the day on a high note. And waiting until the end of the day to eat your most satisfying meal—the one with few limitations—is the best way I know to do that.

It's a balance. For most of us, nighttime is a time to relax and enjoy ourselves, and eating is a part of that. (Cooking is a part of that, too, and of VB6.) Whether it's biologically "correct" to eat your big meal after dark is less important than establishing a diet that doesn't make you crazy by putting you out of touch not only with your entire history but with your friends and your social life.

Here again it's not only the number of calories you eat but also the *type* of calories. Since VB6 allows for animal products at dinner, you'll naturally be consuming a higher concentration of protein and fat at night, and perhaps a portion of something sweet. (More on that on page 102.)

Yet your processed carbohydrate levels will never be high so your glucose won't spike, your insulin won't switch into high gear, and you'll leave the table satisfied. The protein, fat, and fiber will keep your body full until you're ready for bed and the "treat factor" of eating foods you've been avoiding all day long will make you, well, happy. So the need to snack after dinner will be minimized. If you do feel the need to snack, it's time to return to the vegan phase and snack on fruit or nuts.

At night, your low hyper-processed–carb meal probably won't prompt your body to store much—if any—excess glucose as fat. In fact, stored fat may be released from your fat cells and liver (in the form of glycogen) to supply the body with the energy it needs to do its nightly repair work. You might even burn fat while you sleep. (Which, by the way, is also important for proper release of leptin, insulin, and ghrelin. In fact, some studies have shown that a single night of any lost sleep can induce insulin resistance.)

All of this science and theory will help you understand the principles behind VB6, which will help you put it into practice. And that's where we're headed next.

3

The Six Principles
of VB6

I didn't have many solid rules when I started on the path toward VB6; I just knew I wasn't going to eat anything but minimally processed fruits, vegetables, grains, nuts, seeds, and legumes until dinnertime. Now, six years later, VB6 is part philosophy and part plan, with six concrete principles. It is how I—and a growing number of friends, readers, and colleagues—eat routinely, effortlessly, and pleasurably. VB6 has become a way of life for me and others.

One thing we've all learned is that it's important to approach VB6 realistically, so that your expectations are met or exceeded, not dashed. I can't promise miracles; there is no magic bullet for weight loss. But I will say this: If you follow the six principles here, you will lose weight, be healthier, feel energized both physically and mentally, and, to top it all off, you'll help change the world for the better. Not bad.

I'll repeat: VB6 isn't about deprivation. You don't have to give up any of the foods you love. Yes, if you're a junk-food junkie, that has to change, though the occasional "cheat" is fine and even expected. But you don't have to eat any bland or unappealing foods, and the volume of food you eat may even increase. Essentially, you'll be shifting the balance of your diet away from animal products and hyper-processed foods and toward plant foods. This includes *literally* unlimited amounts of most vegetables and all fruits; moderate quantities of beans, whole grains, nuts, and healthy fats; and minimal portions of animal products, processed carbohydrates, alcohol—and anything that qualifies as junk.

Consider these principles as guidelines, not rules: You can—and should—tweak them to fit your life and personality. But remember: They're the backbone of successful and sustainable weight loss and long-term good health. The more closely you follow them, the greater success you will have.

1. EAT FRUIT AND VEGETABLES IN ABUNDANCE

The Standard American Diet (SAD) has little in common with the way people have been eating for millennia, and our health suffers as a result. Foods close to their natural state nourished our ancestors for thousands of years before fast food came on the scene, and still feed many people throughout the Mediterranean, Latin America, Africa, and Asia. Their diets consist mostly of vegetables, whole grains, beans, and fruit, with harder-to-come-by meat, poultry, fish, eggs, and dairy eaten in small portions as garnishes, condiments, or side dishes. (The exceptions are people who live in extremely cold and barren climates, where animal foods and fats necessarily dominate the indigenous diet.) Historically, few people could afford to eat meat frequently or in quantities; meat was for feasts and treats. And it's no coincidence that obesity and related preventable diseases like Type 2 diabetes were scarce until the newfangled SAD began to take over, first in the United States and now around the globe.

This principle—eat fruits and vegetables in abundance—means two things. You can eat almost all fruits and vegetables in unlimited quantities; a few, like legumes, nuts, seeds, whole grains, starchy or fatty vegetables or fruits, and oils, should be eaten more moderately. There's more detail about this on pages 94–102, but for now just know that plant foods will be your go-to foods. Once you increase your vegetable and fruit consumption, the balance of your diet will naturally shift away from animal products and junk.

Remember that fruits and vegetables are full of fiber and water, which is why you can eat a lot of them. (If you eat large amounts of beans, nuts, and whole grains, which are almost as calorie dense [and filling] as animal products, you will likely still lose weight, but more slowly.)

But even after eating until you're full (and fiber and water will fill you up fast), you'll probably feel that familiar urge to snack before it's time for your next meal. And that's fine. There's nothing wrong with snacking, as long as you make the right choices. Grab some fruit, some carrots and celery, or a handful of nuts; if you're at home, toss together a salad or eat last night's leftover vegetables. Snacking only becomes a problem when two dangerous tendencies meet: We eat even though we're not really hungry, and we reach for stuff that contains everything we should try to avoid—the "snack foods" so prevalent in the SAD.

This may sound limited and boring to you, and certainly you'll need variety. But if you start filling your fridge with a mix of leafy vegetables (lettuce, spinach, chard, collards, and kale), cruciferous vegetables (cabbage, broccoli, cauliflower, and Brussels sprouts), fruit-like vegetables (tomatoes, zucchini, eggplant, and winter squash), and root vegetables (beets, turnips, radishes, and carrots), you're going to have plenty of options. You may not like every vegetable you encounter, but you'll find plenty that you do, as you integrate them into your life. Chances are if you favor one in a group, you'll like others. Like spinach or cabbage? Give bok choy a go. Fennel is a flavorful swap for celery; parsnips are like a more intensely flavored carrot. And so on.

Learn about the vegetables that are native to your area and in season, since local produce is fresher and better tasting than stuff that's been shipped halfway around the world. But remember that frozen fruit and vegetables are packed soon after harvest, so in addition to being handy, their quality is often as good as "fresh," since much of what is "fresh" is days or even weeks old by the time you buy it.

Some vegetables are better eaten in moderation: Starchy vegetables like white potatoes are rich in fiber and micronutrients, but they're more akin to grains or beans in calorie density, and are quickly broken down into sugar. So not only will you want to minimize chips and fries (mostly fat anyway), but refrain from making potatoes a major contributor to your diet. Some high-fat fruits and vegetables, like avocados and olives, are great as snacks or alternatives to cheese, but because they're quite calorie dense, it's best to go easy on them. (Still, any time you want to eat an avocado instead of a cheeseburger, that's a fair swap.)

In general, green and orange vegetables are preferable, and you can eat them any time you like. Using a variety of cooking techniques and seasonings helps to keep any diet rich and interesting. If you don't already know, you'll soon learn that anything you can do with fish, poultry, and meat, you can do with vegetables—roasting, broiling, grilling, pan-cooking, and stir-frying, as well as poaching and steaming. And of course you can eat fruit and veggies raw; few animal-based dishes are as easy or as complex as a great salad.

Fruit is a godsend when you're craving something sweet. It even comes in convenient, individually portioned units: Think of apples, pears, bananas, and oranges as nature's original 100-calorie snack packs, and eat a piece whenever you're hungry. (I sometimes need to eat two or even three apples to feel satisfied, and there's nothing wrong with that.) Take advantage not only of seasonally perfect fruit but also of good-quality frozen fruit. Whirl some in the food processor and you get instant sorbet.

Augment fruits and vegetables with whole, unprocessed grains. Brown rice, steel-cut or rolled oats, cornmeal, quinoa, bulgur, wheat berries, hominy (posole), and other whole grains are all fair game, all day long, though in moderation. Real whole-grain bread and whole-grain pasta are part of this category, too (but few commercially available versions of these foods are actually "minimally processed"; see page 45). And remember that white flour, white rice, and other hyper-processed grains are not "whole" and have lost most of their nutritional properties; think of them as treats (more on this in Principle Three on page 75).

You need not be a grain connoisseur; in fact, if you eat a bowl of oatmeal in the morning and switch from white to (true) whole-grain bread, you'll already be ahead of the game. But the more you get into eating whole grains, the more you'll want to explore.

Next on the menu are legumes: chickpeas, lentils, cannellini, kidney, black, pinto, and other beans, split peas, black-eyed peas, and all of their relatives, soybeans—and a zillion others. (Peanuts are technically

FIVE STRATEGIES FOR EATING MORE PLANT FOODS

1. **Buy them.** It may sound silly, but the first step is to actually *shop*. If you've got your supplies lined up, you'll turn to them instead of junk food when you get hungry. And if you load up the fridge with fruits and vegetables—whatever they are—you'll be far more likely to eat them. If you create a detailed eating plan (check out pages 123–126) for breakfast, lunch, snacks, and dinner, you can make sure you have all the necessary ingredients.

2. **Prep vegetables so they're always ready to eat.** When you get home from the store—or whenever you're on the phone, watching TV, or have a few minutes—trim carrots and celery, cut them into sticks, and store them in water in the fridge. Rinse lettuce, tear it into pieces, and stash it in towels in plastic bags or a salad spinner; that way you can make a salad in three minutes. Pre-cook broccoli, cauliflower, or string beans—in boiling water or in the microwave—so they're ready to add to recipes or snack on when you want them. Wash a bunch of fruit and put it in a bowl.

3. **Make big batches of grains and beans every week.** Cooking beans and grains requires virtually no effort, and they keep in the fridge for days or in the freezer indefinitely. If you freeze them in 1-cup portions, they'll hold up well and defrost quickly. (If they don't last all week, good work! Make some more.) Or you can sock away a few different kinds for variety. Once you have them ready to go, salads, soups, and stir-fries come together in an instant.

4. **Step out of your comfort zone.** There's a wide world of vegetables, fruits, grains, beans, and nuts out there; explore it. To avoid getting stuck in a rut, resolve to try at least one new plant every month—you're bound to like and even love some of them. And you'll virtually never run out of options.

5. **Experiment with ways to make vegetables exciting.** Be sure to try other techniques like roasting, grilling, broiling, sautéing, or braising. And don't be afraid of adding some fat (especially olive oil), spices, and/or herbs. Finally, don't forget: An ounce of bacon or Parmesan goes a long way (after 6!).

a legume, though obviously we think of them as nuts.) VB6 becomes a lot easier if you eat beans daily; they're high in protein and fiber, and they're delicious, versatile, and easy to cook in bulk and reheat (see "Building Blocks," page 228). They're filling, too. And beans' well-publicized and widely mocked digestive side effects go away in almost everyone who eats them regularly.

Finally, nuts. Crunchy, nutritious, beloved, and a way better choice than snack foods like chips. Nuts are also super calorie dense, so you shouldn't eat them with abandon, but an ounce of them buries an ounce of chips for both nutrition and satisfaction. You can also use nuts when you're cooking to add both crunch and flavor to grain dishes and salads. You'll probably also come to depend on peanut butter and other nut butters.

One final word about all of these plant foods: In recent years, everything from oats to pomegranates to walnuts has been heralded as a "superfood" that fights disease and promotes good health. In truth, every whole plant food contains beneficial micronutrients, but no single plant gives you all the nutrients you need. So ignore overblown marketing claims and focus instead on eating a variety of plants. Period.

2. EAT FEWER ANIMAL PRODUCTS

Along with eating more plants, this is fundamental to VB6, from both nutritional and environmental standpoints. Of all the changes you can make to your diet, eating fewer animal products has the most dramatic impact on the health of the planet—and a huge impact on your personal health as well.

Eating fewer animal products is the inevitable future. There is not enough land, water, energy, or mineral resources for the earth's billions to consume animal products at the rate we do, and the knowledge that we as individuals can take such a simple step to affect the fate of the planet is extremely empowering. For example, if we each ate the equivalent of three fewer cheeseburgers a week, we'd cancel out the effects of all the SUVs in the country. That's the road we need to be on.

There are other reasons, of course: If you believe that animals deserve decent lives relatively free of suffering, it's time to eat less (or no) industrially produced meat. The term "factory farming" is for real; animals are produced as if they were widgets, with little to no care for their welfare or the quality of the product.

So unless you're a vegan, or a self-sufficient farmer, or spend a *lot* of time and money buying products from local farmers, you're complicit to some degree. I am; it's nearly impossible to live in the United States and not be. But VB6 helps you significantly limit your participation in this morally questionable system.

Then, of course, there's health: Eating fewer animal products is key to avoiding chronic disease, because while they're good sources of protein and certain micronutrients, they're high in saturated fat

THREE STRATEGIES FOR EATING FEWER ANIMAL FOODS

1. **Buy half as much meat, and make it better meat.** Think of eating meat as the indulgence it is. The average American eats about a half-pound of meat a day; one of the first steps in VB6 is reducing that amount. Any reduction is better than none, and more reduction is better than some. At the same time, use better, more sustainable animal products. They're more expensive, yes, but since you'll be buying smaller quantities, the budget won't change much. Remember, most international cuisines use meat as a condiment, garnish, or treat.

2. **Get over the meat-as-main-course mentality.** I'm not suggesting you put an eggplant in the center of the plate (though you certainly could), but that you tweak the proportions of meat to plants in your diet. Build your meals around what were once called "sides"—vegetables, of course, but also rice, grains, beans, noodles, and pasta. Meat is a treat, not the main event, and 3 ounces will satisfy your craving as well as 8 ounces, once you change the balance on your plate.

3. **Cook plants as you would meat.** They're just as versatile and convenient, and many legumes, nuts, and whole grains are good sources of protein. Anything you can do with meat you can do with vegetables— sometimes even more. Check out the recipes beginning on page 136.

and cholesterol, calorie dense, and often tainted by antibiotics. Until the SAD became the norm—with its quarter-pound cheeseburgers, 16-ounce steaks, cheese-stuffed pizzas, and four-egg omelets—we had not been so fat nor had such chronic health issues. It's not that these animal-based foods are inherently bad, but that they're produced badly and we're eating them morning, noon, and night. Eat higher quality animal products and fewer of them, and many things change for the better.

When you move away from the meat-as-a-main mentality and start to build your meals around plants, you quickly begin to think of animal products as a form of seasoning. I'm not talking about forgoing meat entirely, but about shifting the balance; you still enjoy the taste and get the satisfaction you crave, but in a healthier, more balanced and more sustainable way. Make the choice: No supplemental grilled chicken on that lunchtime salad, thanks. Pass the chickpeas.

Finally, a word about fish: It's undeniably good for you, a mostly lean source of protein with lots of beneficial unsaturated fat. And wild fish is as "natural" and "organic" as it gets. The same, however, cannot be said of farm-raised fish (which are routinely fed lots of antibiotics, like other farm-raised animals), and there are concerns about toxins in many wild fish. Furthermore, fishing of big fish—the kind we most like to eat—has yet to be managed in a sustainable way. Purely from a health perspective, you can eat fish with more confidence than other animal products, but you have to be pretty careful if you don't want to contribute to the dwindling numbers of many species. And fish, like other animal foods, should be reserved for after six o'clock.

3. EAT (ALMOST) NO JUNK FOOD

You know this already. Eating more plants and fewer animals is a critical part of VB6, but reducing—even abandoning—your consumption of hyper-processed and junk foods is just as imperative.

You know what they are: Foods that are unrecognizable as coming from their source (like Pringles), contain ingredients you've never heard of (like energy bars), are thought of as quick meals (Hot Pockets, to name just one), are ultra high-calorie (ice cream—I know, you need it now and then, but not every night), are nutritionally useless or even damaging (soda), and so on down the list of hyper-processed snacks, drinks, and fast food. Like pornography, junk might be tough to define but you know it when you see it.

That said, is there a difference between white pasta and nacho cheese chips? Absolutely. Processed food isn't *necessarily* junk food. Just as animal products are seen as treats, so too are pasta, white rice, and real white bread. They should be eaten sparingly, but they're also traditional food made of real ingredients. It's okay to indulge in that plate of pasta now and then, but that microwave dinner with thirty-four ingredients can hardly be considered food. And soon you won't think of it that way anymore, and you'll be better off for it.

There is a lot of personal judgment at play here. Cured and smoked meats, cheese, processed animal foods, alcohol—all these traditional processed foods must be considered treats. You can indulge in some amount of each, even daily, but remember that a grating of Parmesan or a piece of Brie (three ingredients, one of which is salt, another milk) is hardly in the same category as processed cheese spread from a can (over a dozen ingredients, many of them chemicals).

It's fairly safe to say that foods with more than five ingredients—an arbitrary number, but a decent guide—count as hyper-processed. (Sadly, many ingredients don't even make it onto food labels, and of course restaurants aren't required to list the components of their menu items, so you need to use your judgment—or go out less.) Once you get to the point where the ingredient list is a paragraph long, what you're eating isn't food so much as a "food product," likely made up of a host of undesirable ingredients.

So pay attention to labels. If a food contains so many ingredients that the side of the box is a block of print, and many of those ingredients are chemical compounds, put it back on the shelf. Stick with real foods. The good news is, if you're eating mostly plants, you won't have to worry too much about this!

Relying on hyper-processed food is a habit that can be broken. You can blame our dependency on the fast pace of modern society, the desire for convenience, Big Food profit-mongers with astronomical market-

FIVE SURE WAYS TO CUT OUT THE JUNK

1. **Don't buy it.** It doesn't get much simpler than that. If you don't keep junk in the house, you're a lot less likely to eat it. Spend your money on vegetables and fruit and small amounts of good-quality animal foods.

2. **Make healthy snacking convenient.** Giving in to junk is usually a matter of desperation: I'm hungry, I'm tired, I'm busy—whatever—but I don't have easy access to good food, so I grab what I can. (And then I regret it.) Keeping a stash of healthy snacks on hand eliminates this problem. Whether it's a bag of nuts, trail mix, fruit, cut-up vegetables, or a bag of popcorn (preferably your own), thinking ahead will save you from a trip to the vending machine and the subsequent wish that you'd had a banana instead. Small changes like carrying fruit to work every day can have a big impact on your life.

3. **Cut out takeout.** Or at least limit it drastically. Fast food can undermine your best intentions. Though there is a spectrum that ranges from good to horrible, with everything in between, there are also plenty of tricks the food industry uses to make something seem healthful when in reality it's filled with fat and sugar. (And it's best to avoid drive-thrus altogether, since you can't see what you're ordering and it's hard to ask questions.)

4. **Bring lunch to work.** The workplace can be stressful and the junk food socially compelling (think of all those birthday cakes!). Too often we grab burgers and chips because we have no alternative. It's far better to eat food that you thought about in advance, even if that means nibbling all day. And recent research bears this out: People who eat food from home at the office lost more weight than those who don't.

5. **Read labels.** Can't say this enough: If it takes you as long to figure out what's in the package as it does to eat it, just put it down and walk away.

ing budgets, or just the appealing (some would say addictive) nature of these foods. For all of those reasons Americans have been conditioned to grab a bag of chips or a candy bar instead of reaching for an apple or a handful of almonds. It's literally killing us.

4. COOK AT HOME AS MUCH AS POSSIBLE

Changing to VB6 involves cooking, which might sound daunting. But I'm not talking about restaurant-style cooking, or the kind of competitive cooking you see on television, but about good home cooking: fast, simple, easy, enjoyable. All it takes is a little practice and a little planning. I've spent literally decades writing about ways to make home cooking as easy and streamlined as possible, and I promise that cooking is an enjoyable and rewarding part of VB6.

But fun is a side benefit. What matters most is that when you cook, you know what you're eating. You'll be in charge of the content of your meals and snacks so you'll easily and automatically shift away from unhealthy carbohydrates, fat, and protein. Cooking is also the easiest way to control the quantity of food you consume: You know exactly how much of every ingredient you use and eat.

You'll also control the quality. Fast food is cheap because it begins with ingredients of the lowest possible quality. (Think about that, because it's true, and ask yourself if that's what you want to routinely put in your body.) You, on the other hand, will start with high-quality ingredients, and you'll cook them with real seasonings. Even if you're used to oversalted, oversweetened, super-fatty junk, I promise you will soon develop a taste for simple cooking. Your food will taste good because your ingredients will be fresh and high quality. It's a no-brainer.

Good cooking makes people happy. It's a great way to unwind; easy, repetitive tasks like chopping and stirring can help you calm down and focus on the moment. And cooking (and sitting down at a real table) has social benefits: It helps you to connect and spend time with friends and loved ones, and appears to have protective benefits as well. Kids who eat regular family dinners are less likely to abuse drugs or develop eating disorders than kids who don't.

Furthermore, the more you cook, the better it gets. As you familiarize yourself with ingredients, you'll come to recognize the signs of good, fresh food: the gentle give when you press on a ripe tomato, the

FIVE EASY WAYS TO GET COOKING

1. **Get equipped.** You don't need a ton of equipment to cook well, but you do need sharp knives, a cutting board, a skillet, a large pot, a colander, a strainer, a few mixing bowls, and some baking dishes. If you're on a budget, look for used equipment, which is usually just fine.

2. **Stock your pantry.** If you have the basics, you'll be far more likely to cook. You can stock your pantry all at once (it probably won't cost more than $100 or so), or you can buy ingredients as you need them. Check out The VB6 Pantry on page 129.

3. **Shop.** Often. Buy fresh produce once or twice a week, more if you have time. If you have vegetables and fruit around, you'll cook with them.

4. **Prepare ingredients ahead of time.** This is touched upon in Principle One, and there are more specific ideas beginning with Chapter 6 (page 127). In short, when you have a moment, do a kitchen task. It'll make cooking easier at dinnertime.

5. **Don't sweat it.** "Perfect" is the enemy of "good," especially in the kitchen; don't get hung up on doing everything just so. You'll make mistakes, but you'll also learn to improvise to compensate for ingredients or skills, or even time that you don't have. The recipes here are simple enough for beginners, with variations for more advanced cooks to explore, and I've included lots of one-dish meals that streamline preparation. Trust me: It's rare that the results will be less delicious than whatever you were going to bring home from the drive-thru or supermarket.

briminess of fresh fish, the snap of green beans. You'll learn to appreciate the better flavor of high-quality meat and chicken, making it easier to avoid the factory-farmed stuff.

This is not about low-fat, low-salt, or low-carb cooking. In fact, my recipes often contain healthy amounts of both fat and carbohydrates, and I'm extremely liberal with my use of salt, which is a crucial addition to make food taste good. (Do you know why much fast food tastes "better" than much "healthy" food? Salt!) But I don't use nearly as much salt as food manufacturers, who must oversalt their foods (even ones that don't taste salty) to make them palatable. (Nor do I have high blood pressure, which appears to be a valid and critical reason to limit your use of salt.) In other words, I don't worry about the amount of salt I add to food in the kitchen because it's never excessive, and I don't think you should, either, unless your doctor tells you otherwise. Undersalting is a minor tragedy.

In the real world, you won't be able to make every meal from scratch, and that's okay. But if you make cooking a priority, and reserve restaurants and takeout for treats, you'll see the benefits pretty quickly: You'll lose weight and feel better, both because you're putting wholesome ingredients and less junk in your body, and because you are actively nourishing yourself and your loved ones.

5. CONSIDER QUALITY OVER QUANTITY

Once you're eating more plants, fewer animal products, and nearly no junk, you'll be eating healthier, better-quality food and fewer calories. But the only way to stay committed is to make sure the food you're eating is at least as enjoyable as the food you're giving up, and what you buy will in part determine your success on VB6. When you reduce your intake of animal products and processed foods, you'll need to replace those foods with the best-quality food you can afford.

Does this mean you should only buy organic fruits and vegetables? No. Are frozen or canned vegetables forbidden? No. Are locally sourced, sustainable meats the only option? No. But the details are nuanced.

We spend a trillion dollars a year on food, but it's only 9.4 percent of our expendable income, the lowest percentage of any country on record. Yet what has cheap food done for us? What is the real cost of cheap food? What are the health costs of cheap food?

You already know the answers to those questions. That's why you're changing your diet.

Good quality is often more expensive, but not always: Fresh produce in season can be quite inexpensive. And frozen produce (which is often a more nutritious and flavorful option than "fresh" out-of-season produce) may also be less expensive than fresh, with the added benefit of eliminating some prep work.

FOUR WAYS TO EAT HIGHER QUALITY FOOD

1. **Spend a little more on a few select items.** Pick and choose where you want to pay extra and where you want to save. There are two possible strategies here: If it's something you enjoy a lot and eat frequently, it might be worth the expense; conversely, if it's a rare treat, maybe you should spend more on it. These strategies are not mutually exclusive.

2. **Know when to buy fresh and when to turn to frozen.** I don't expect you to become an agricultural expert, but it's easy enough to tell what's in season. Obviously, tropical fruits are grown near few readers of this book, but you're still going to enjoy them whenever you can. On the other hand, in January you're probably better off with frozen green beans or corn than hunting down "fresh" that comes from another hemisphere.

3. **Explore international markets.** The markets of immigrant groups or of people who are less assimilated, food-wise (and who therefore may be eating less of the SAD), are the best places to shop for interesting produce, legumes, and spices. Check out Southeast Asian, Chinese, Japanese, Indian, Korean, Mexican, and South American markets, for example, and don't be intimidated: You're a customer!

4. **Waste as little as possible.** Throwing food away is literally money down the drain. Think of ways to "repurpose" whatever vegetables, salads, grains, or beans you have from dinner the night before into the next day's lunch, even if you just use it as sandwich filling or toss it into salad.

Undeniably, well-raised meat, poultry, dairy, and eggs often cost more than their factory-farmed counterparts, and they should: There's more work in producing them. In fact, for farmers to make a decent living and respect their animals, land, and even consumers, most good food should be priced even higher than it is now.

But VB6 means that you'll be buying less meat than you did and using it in smaller quantities. And since legumes, grains, fruits, and vegetables are generally less expensive than animal products, your food budget could well go down, especially if you eat out less often. You can buy a pound of beans that will feed you for days for less than you'd pay for a Quarter Pounder with Cheese. And improving your health is obviously a smart investment.

6. SEE YOUR WEIGHT AS JUST ONE COMPONENT OF GOOD HEALTH

VB6 is not a "lose weight fast!" diet. The changes outlined in these pages have more to do with living a healthy life than with having a reed-thin body.

And just as marketing has redefined food (high fructose corn syrup, anyone?), it's warped our notion of what constitutes a "good" body. We've gotten more than 20 percent fatter over the past fifty years, yet our physical ideal as expressed by the media has become thinner. I don't know anyone who doesn't think he or she needs to lose at least 5 pounds, regardless of present size, and if you're comfortable with your body (congrats!), you're an anomaly.

But healthy bodies come in all shapes and sizes. There is no single "ideal" weight applicable to more than one person; depending on your metabolism, your genetics, and your body composition, your ideal weight might be 10 or even 20 pounds heavier than that of someone else of the same height and gender.

Few of us are destined to look like models, and we won't, even if we starve ourselves, because deprivation dieting doesn't work: The majority of dieters yo-yo, gaining their weight back and then some. What is achievable by almost everyone in this country is a healthy diet that will moderate your weight, and VB6 moves you in that direction the moment you start it.

Then there is exercise: Our sedentary lifestyle has contributed nearly as much to our collective health crisis as our diet, and reversing the situation will require not only eating better but also moving more. And the benefits of exercise for physical, mental, and psychological well-being are immense. Being strong and fit increases your will and your determination, and therefore can play a big part in keeping you committed to VB6.

Anyone can find an enjoyable activity; you just have to try some. And exercise can be almost any activity: a walk; a run; a bike ride; a weight-lifting session; a yoga, Pilates, or step class; or the stairs instead of the elevator. (Even cooking, to some extent!) Any physical activity will improve your health and make you feel better.

FIVE TIPS FOR FEELING TRULY HEALTHY

1. **Don't let the media decide how you should look.** Remind yourself that almost every magazine image has been retouched to within an inch of its life, and that the vast majority of human beings don't look anything like models.

2. **Don't obsess over the scale.** It's harder to attach your self-worth to a number when you don't know what that number is, and by avoiding the scale you avoid that number. By not focusing on how much your weight has changed in the last two hours, it's easier to focus on how you actually feel. Which may actually be pretty good. (You might, however, want to monitor your weight every week or so, to make sure you're going in the right direction, or remaining stable if that's your goal.)

3. **Wear clothes that fit and flatter.** No good has ever come of buying pants that are too tight in hopes that you'll lose weight and be able to fit into them. Wear clothes that fit and make you feel confident, and pack away clothes that are too small until you're ready to try them on again.

4. **Treat yourself the way you treat others.** You probably don't judge other people's bodies nearly as harshly as you judge your own. Would you tell your best friend or your mother that she's disgusting and unattractive because of the size and shape of her body? If you wouldn't say it about someone else's body, don't say it about yours.

5. **Focus on the holistic benefits of exercise.** Beyond feeling stronger and healthier, even moderate activity like walking or gardening can help you relax, sleep better, and boost your mood.

And once you start exercising regularly, you'll feel better about your body and never want to stop. (Exercise is addictive. Literally.) You'll improve your endurance, speed, strength, and/or flexibility; you'll see that you can be fit, healthy, and capable regardless of how much you weigh.

Some studies have shown that exercise might not help you lose weight; after all, it makes you hungrier, prompting you to eat enough to offset the calories you've burned. (That's been my experience!) But the benefits of exercise outweigh mere weight loss: Regular exercise promotes cardiovascular health, prevents diabetes, delays the onset of dementia and Alzheimer's disease, keeps your bones and joints strong, and reduces the risk of cancer. Exercise is for fitness and health; weight loss comes from eating fewer calories. The combination of a good exercise routine and VB6 will give you both.

Most diet book authors do their best to convince you that your body isn't good enough, that fat is a moral failure, and that "success" depends fully on how many pounds you lose. The typical diet also makes false promises of radical weight loss and leads you to believe that if you don't achieve that, it's because you're not disciplined enough.

But if you're eating well and exercising, and your weight is 5, 10, 15, or more pounds above what you had considered ideal, you might question your expectations. Are you letting unrealistic standards determine how you feel about yourself?

Here's what I propose instead: Set your goal as overall improved health. Follow the VB6 principles and plan. Use the recipes to help you avoid junk food. Exercise regularly. You'll be healthier and lose weight in the bargain.

TWEAK THE PRINCIPLES SO THEY WORK FOR YOU

At this point, you have all the information, all the tools, and, I hope, all the reasons for why you should make this lifestyle change. That doesn't mean it will be easy. What matters is that you're excited to make a commitment to yourself to go VB6.

Not all of these principles will work for everyone in their most extreme form. For some, eliminating meat altogether will be a cinch; for others, cutting out bacon in the morning might be a big step. The point is that both approaches are equally valuable because they're changes in the right direction. It's important to put VB6—and your progress following these principles—on a continuum. Unlike so many diets, this isn't an all-or-nothing proposition. You can make changes incrementally, and your level of commitment can be plotted on a spectrum ranging from extremely devoted to grudgingly enthusiastic. It's about moving in the right direction; at one end of the spectrum is the worst level of the SAD; at the other is a hyper-committed vegan living on unprocessed plants. Almost all of us fall somewhere in the middle; the most important aspect of VB6 is to move in the right direction, the direction of a plant-based diet. It doesn't matter if you never get all the way there: Just keep moving.

To make sure that VB6 can work for everyone at every point of the spectrum, I provide one basic, structured VB6 28-Day Plan that can be easily adapted to your specific style. The next chapter goes into more detail about this, but this is the gist: Depending on what kind of eater you are, you may respond better to a more structured program or thrive with more flexibility. The various profiles in the next part of the book are designed specifically to make sure VB6 can work for you in a way that makes you happy and keeps you committed.

Of course, even the most dedicated among us is going to have bad days, maybe even bad weeks, but in the grand scheme of things, falling off the wagon isn't the end of the world. Anyone who exercises or has other activities that require self-discipline knows that there are good periods and less good ones. You might, for example, plan to exercise five times a week and hit just four, and some weeks even three—or none. That doesn't mean you're not exercising; it means you're not per-fect, which you probably knew already.

It's the same with adopting a VB6 diet: Just because you lapse for a meal, or even a month, it doesn't mean you should beat yourself up and call it quits. On the contrary, part of the beauty of this way of eating and living is that you can give in to cravings once in a while—go out for a wildly decadent dinner, take a week off while you're on vacation if you like—as long as you find your way back. Remember, this isn't just a four-week crash regimen; it's a lifelong plan.

PART TWO

MAKING VB6 WORK FOR YOU

4

Eating VB6

I call VB6 a "diet" only reluctantly. I prefer to describe it as a journey toward change, complete with twists and turns—including some very inevitable, very human backtracking—that ultimately leads to a better life. Along the way, you'll learn to think about food differently. You'll make real food your first choice; you'll begin to see vegetables, fruits, and other plant foods in a new light, and cooking and eating with family and friends will take on a brighter, healthier character. You'll order a little differently at restaurants (this will feel odd at first, but not for long) and navigate parties with a fresh perspective. With every day, you'll be gaining health, losing weight (or maintaining it), feeling renewed energy, and changing your outlook.

THE PATH TO LASTING CHANGE

Regardless of how drastic or subtle these changes will be for you, it's easier to make change—to break unwanted habits and establish new patterns—with a strategy. That's the experience of the tens of millions of people who have stopped smoking, and it's been confirmed by research. While anyone can try quitting cold turkey, most people are more likely to be successful if they plan their change because change—

any change—is a process, and it's one that works on both conscious and unconscious levels.

The path to making sustainable, lasting change involves four phases:

- In Phase 1, you *decide* that a change is necessary and are motivated to explore new behavior.

- In Phase 2, you *plan* and start to think about how to achieve that change.

- In Phase 3, you *act*, putting the plan in motion.

- And in Phase 4, you *maintain* the plan and change your behavior for good.

Decide. Plan. Act. Maintain. If you look back on any lasting change you've made in your life, you'll likely see that it followed this pattern. And this book follows these same four steps.

Deciding that you're ready for change is the all-important first step toward action. Not until you've acknowledged that there is an issue will you seriously begin thinking about the benefits of a new course. Admitting that there's a part of life that no longer feels comfortable, or might even be harmful—even if it's a habit you enjoy (or claim to enjoy)—takes energy and openness to explore: How big a priority is this change? Do you feel fully committed or resistant? Are you afraid to give up comfortable behaviors?

This sounds familiar, I'm sure. After all, you're reading this book because you've already come to some kind of realization, and in doing so you've demonstrated your motivation: You're well on your way to *deciding* to make change.

The discussion of the Standard American Diet (SAD) and the science behind VB6 in Chapters 1 and 2 should have given you ammunition for increasing your motivation to make a change in the way you eat and live, and (I hope) helped you understand ways you can adjust and improve your diet. If you ever forget why you started this journey, that evidence can be a touchstone to help get you back on track.

After you decide to alter your behavior, it's time to contemplate what has to happen for this change to take place—what can remain constant in your life and what must be adjusted for your new idea to take hold. You start Phase 2: to *plan*. Becoming familiar with the six fundamental principles of VB6 helped you make the transition from deciding to planning. The theories and tips outlined in Chapter 3 were designed to help you envision how reaching your goal would play out in real life—and the possible outcomes. I encourage you to revisit the Six Principles whenever you need to step back from day-to-day events—and especially setbacks—and focus instead on the big picture.

You've decided that the way you eat—this essential part of the way you live, this daily routine that is so much a part of you—is no longer working, on one or more levels. You're motivated to transform something you do out of habit, love, boredom, stress, and likely a combination, into something more positive, something that is actually better—for you. And you've had a glimpse of what your life will be like when you adopt the VB6 way of eating. The next step is to *act*.

Phases 3 and 4 of this journey are not easy: Changing how you eat is a big deal. We eat to live, of course, but the rituals and gestures surrounding how we do it are well-ingrained habits, ways we establish familiarity and comfort, things we gravitate toward eagerly and repetitively. Think about your favorite meals ("I love my mom's lasagna," or "My favorite lunch is the roast beef sub with extra mayo"), snacks that you grab almost thoughtlessly (nachos at your favorite Mexican restaurant, a box of cookies when you get home), or indulgences that bring us some sort of solace (for tens of millions of us, ice cream).

Lifelong patterns don't go away without awareness and discipline. But creating and maintaining new habits can be rewarding; setting and achieving goals are challenges unique to human experience, and even *attempting* to reach them can give you hope and encouragement that will enrich your life. There's a reason that the journey is said to be more important than the destination, and that's why it's important to view VB6 not only as beneficial but as exciting.

So, feel the excitement begin and let it build as you put your plan into action and start reaping the enormous benefits of the changes you're going to make.

Putting the plan into action means considering a different and more specific set of questions: What, how, and when will you begin VB6?

How can you make it easier on yourself? Will you ease into it, or would you rather plunge right in? What are your goals? Are they realistic? How long are you willing to wait to see results? Acting on your decision to change requires optimism, dedication, and a sense of confidence and empowerment: the feeling that you can *do this*, and even when you bump into obstacles along the way, *you'll stick with your plan.*

Change loves company, so if you can rally family members, co-workers, or friends to do VB6 with you, all the better. The complicity is helpful in more ways than one: You share experiences—eating, cooking, planning, talking about meals, successes and difficulties—and you can support, encourage, and inspire each other.

In fact, VB6 is both exciting and pleasurable. You'll discover new foods as you abandon or de-emphasize those that are attacking your well-being. And you'll feel good almost instantly. As each day passes, you'll forge new eating patterns: You'll be seeing food differently and enjoying it more.

The most difficult, and longest phase, of course, is sustaining the change, making your new diet permanent; much of the balance of this book is filled with practical, day-to-day information and recipes that will help you do just that.

But before I get into the nuts and bolts of eating and cooking VB6, I would be remiss not to touch on the emotional component of committing to this lifestyle. When I started eating VB6, I was pleasantly surprised to find that it seemed little more than a fun challenge. There'd be a day here or there when I couldn't believe how much I craved good, crusty white bread with lunch (and sometimes I succumbed), and afternoons when it seemed impossible to live without a slice of pizza (and sometimes I gave in to that, also), but for the most part I felt as if I were on a voyage of discovery.

It soon became more than that, though, because VB6 is self-reinforcing. As I said before, I quickly lost weight (and have now kept it off for six years, something I doubt I'd be reporting if I'd gone on a conventional diet) and saw the numbers on my blood work improve.

That wasn't all, though. As you'll no doubt have noticed, my rules for VB6 are quite strict: no animal products before six o'clock, but also no white flour, white rice, pasta, no junk food—and no sugar at all. (Okay, full disclosure: Sometimes I put sugar in my coffee.) But my "rules" for after 6 P.M. were nonexistent. I allowed myself to eat, literally, whatever I felt like. But as the months went by, I found myself eating fewer animal products and in smaller amounts, even at dinner, relying more and more on plants. And although sugar and refined flour were technically "allowed" after 6 o'clock, cutting out those items throughout the day made me less interested in having sweets after dinner. (I hardly ever eat dessert now—not even once a week—though I do sometimes have a little chocolate in the afternoon.) I developed new habits, and as a result my cravings actually changed.

And my eating habits have stayed that way. Yes, there are splurge nights when I eat a steak or pass dishes around the table at a restaurant until all the food is gone. But the majority of nights are a midway point between how I used to eat and how I now eat during the day: essentially, a flexitarian approach. (You'll see that the recipes in the dinner section reflect this approach, neither vegan nor full-on carnivore.) All of which is to say VB6 is easier to sustain than you might imagine.

Undoubtedly, you'll be attracted by junk food, burgers, and pizza, day in and day out. The sensation of passing a McDonald's and craving a fix, even when you're not hungry (yes, I know that feeling), is a sign of how well and thoroughly we've been manipulated by Big Food. These aren't nutritional cravings, of course, but learned ones. And there'll be days when you give in to old habits. But as long as you feel committed, and remember that VB6 is a new way of eating for life—not a short-term fix—that you can pick up again right where you left off, you'll be fine. With this diet there is no beginning, middle, or end.

Sometimes I think of it this way: I'm a runner, and have been for nearly forty years. And there have been times, many of them, when I didn't lace up my shoes for a week, or even more. That matters, but it doesn't make me a non-runner; exercise is a part of who I am, and one of the ways I identify myself, whether I'm training for my next marathon or squeezing in three miles a week.

And that's how VB6 is, too. Once you commit to it, it'll become part of you, even if you stray for a meal—or for a week. (Your weight will tell you if you've strayed too far, even if you don't use a scale.)

If you're ready to make this change, then I believe you'll happily choose to sustain this way of eating for the rest of your life. And, unquestionably, you'll benefit from it.

THE VB6 FOOD GROUPS

Now comes the fun part: what you'll actually eat. One of the best things about VB6 is that it encourages you to enjoy a wide and delicious variety of foods, in generous portions. Your choices are broad—infinite, really, but clearly divided into three groups: Unlimited Foods, Flexible Foods, and Treats. These categories are derived from the science behind metabolism, calorie density, and glycemic index described in Chapter 2 and the Six Principles outlined in Chapter 3. And if you pay attention to nothing *but* these simple distinctions—and once you see some examples, it will become obvious where a given food belongs on this spectrum—you will have great success with VB6. There's nothing more you need to worry about or keep track of. Learn these distinctions, and you'll have all you need to navigate the supermarket, your kitchen, a restaurant, or the office.

In the course of thirty-plus years of teaching how to shop and cook, I've learned that thinking of ingredients in discrete groups inspires confidence and fosters flexibility. In the context of VB6, these groupings will guide how you eat *for a lifetime*, without counting points or calories. When you use these groups to make food choices, you'll inevitably reduce the overall number of calories in your meals, especially the kinds of calories responsible for weight gain.

Remember: Being Vegan Before 6 requires only that you shift the balance of what you eat, not eliminate foods entirely.

UNLIMITED FOODS

Fruit, most vegetables, most condiments, and all herbs and spices form the foundation of your diet. Eat freely and luxuriously from this category.

VEGETABLES
Vegetables are without question the healthiest and most expansive family of foods. All offer vital nutrients and the best nutrient-to-calorie ratio, most provide lots of fiber, and they come in a variety of colors,

textures, and flavors to keep you interested and satisfied from one meal to the next. If you haven't explored all of the types on this list—which is by no means exhaustive—now is your chance. And it doesn't matter whether they're raw or cooked: Just Eat Them. Here's a hardly exhaustive but representative rundown (a few exceptions are among the Flexible Foods listed below):

- **Cabbage-like vegetables and greens:** All lettuces and salad greens, spinach, watercress, cabbage, broccoli, cauliflower, Brussels sprouts, broccoli raab, bok choy (and other Asian greens), kale, collards, chard, escarole, dandelion, chicory, endive
- **Nightshades (the fruits of the vegetable world):** Eggplant, bell peppers, chiles, tomatoes, tomatillos
- **Stalk or stem vegetables:** Celery, fennel, asparagus, mushrooms, artichokes, cardoons, kohlrabi, cactus
- **Edible-pod legumes:** Green and wax beans, snow peas, snap peas

- **Root vegetables and tubers:** Carrots, radishes, beets, celery root, turnips, rutabaga, parsnips, sweet potatoes, yams, jícama
- **Summer squashes:** Zucchini, yellow, pattypan
- **Winter squashes:** Pumpkin, butternut, acorn, spaghetti, kabocha, delicata
- **Aromatics:** Onions, leeks, garlic, scallions, shallots, ginger
- **Sprouts:** Alfalfa, lentil, wheat, radish, soy and bean sprouts
- **Sea vegetables:** Seaweeds and sea beans

FRUIT

This is where VB6 differs from most diets: You can eat as much fruit as you'd like (again, the few exceptions are noted among the Flexible Foods listed below). With its fiber and natural sweetness fruit will fill you up and satisfy your sweet tooth, often helping you resist the temptation to reach for a candy bar or bowl of ice cream. And that's really the point: Fruit will always be better for you than junk food, and it's a fantastic stopgap to get you to six o'clock, when you can indulge a bit. I've even found that the habit of starting a meal with a little fruit salad or a half-grapefruit—as many moms (including mine) did in the '60s—prevents me from overindulging on the entrée or dessert. Fruit in season is always tastiest, but frozen (unsweetened) fruit is also fine. I know you know how to recognize it, but here's a reminder of the options:

- **Citrus:** Oranges, grapefruit, lemons, limes, tangerines, mandarins, clementines, tangelos
- **Melons:** Watermelon, cantaloupe, honeydew, casaba

- **Stone and tree fruit:** Apples, pears, peaches, nectarines, apricots, plums, cherries, figs
- **Tropicals:** Bananas and plantains, mango, pineapple, papaya, kiwi

CONDIMENTS AND SEASONINGS

Not only do they keep other foods vibrant and interesting, the choices on this list contain no sugar and have low calorie densities. Some, especially herbs and spices, contain beneficial micronutrients not found elsewhere, but for the most part these ingredients don't have much of anything except flavor. I use them liberally in my recipes—sample them on their own and decide which you like best; each has the potential to make something as simple as steamed vegetables memorable.

- **Salt and pepper:** I don't fuss over these; use whatever you like. And as long as you're cooking your own food (and don't have high blood pressure), feel free to salt to taste.

- **Fresh herbs:** Handfuls of chopped parsley, basil, mint, chives, or cilantro; smaller amounts of everything else.

- **Dried herbs:** The best are oregano, marjoram, sage, thyme, and rosemary; the rest have little flavor.

- **Vinegars:** I like them all, but sherry is my favorite.

- **Mustard:** Coarse and Dijon-style; I use both. (Avoid those with added sugar, like honey mustard.)

- **Salsa (without fat):** Make your own (page 240) or get the good stuff in jars, not cans.

- **Hot sauces:** Srirachas and sambals included.

- **Pickles:** Any vegetable, as long as the brine is unsweetened.

- **Soy sauce:** Nothing adds savory flavor faster; buy only the real stuff fermented from soy and wheat, not those made of colored water.

- **Miso:** Any color; thinned with a little water, this is an instant sauce.

- **Spices and spice blends:** All of them, but pimentón (smoked paprika), curry and chili powders, garam masala, jerk seasoning, and fines herbes are among my favorites.

- **Worcestershire and fish sauce (nam pla):** These aren't technically vegan, but from a VB6 perspective the amount of animal products they contain is trivial.

FLEXIBLE FOODS

These foods provide important nutrients, but are generally more calorie dense than fruits, vegetables, condiments, and seasonings. Eat them sparingly at breakfast, lunch, or in snacks; after 6 P.M. you have more latitude with the foods in this category. They are the following:

BEANS

Beans ("legumes" is the name for this entire category) are a great source of protein, and since they're loaded with fiber, they're quite filling. There are so many that if you ate a different type every week, you wouldn't get through them all in ten years. You can cook your own (see page 236 for a recipe), or use convenient canned or frozen kinds (see page 238 for some tips). And they're great hot, cold, alone, or with other food. My personal favorites are white beans, lentils, and chickpeas, but I eat them all, usually daily. (Once you eat them frequently, their well-reported gas-causing properties disappear.) Here's a short (and incomplete) list:

- **Lentils**
- **Cannellini, navy, great northern, and other white beans**
- **Chickpeas** (garbanzos)
- **Black beans**
- **Black-eyed peas**
- **Lima and gigante beans**
- **Kidney beans** (and their immature version, flageolets)
- **Pinto and cranberry beans**
- **Fava beans**
- **Soybeans**
- **Mung beans**

WHOLE GRAINS

The important distinction here is that you rely on whole grains—not their highly processed "white" counterparts. Your first choice should be whole grains in their minimally milled form (these appear at the top of this list). Foods made by processing whole grains into flour are still considered Flexible, but know that your body converts them to glucose more quickly than it will the grains in their unrefined state. There's a lot more about this starting on page 44, but in a nutshell, whole grains contain the fiber and protein you need to stay satisfied in the long haul and are more nutritious. (I'm not saying you can't ever have white bread or pasta; you'll find those foods listed among the Treats.) This is an incomplete list, and I urge you to seek out even more; see page 235 for a recipe that shows you how to cook them all.

- **Brown rice** (all kinds)
- **Bulgur**
- **Cornmeal and polenta**
- **Oats** (all kinds except instant)
- **Quinoa**
- **Cracked wheat**
- **Wheat and rye berries**
- **Wild rice**
- **Buckwheat groats and kasha**
- **Farro**
- **Barley** (hulled not pearled)
- **Hominy and grits**
- **Kamut**
- **Millet**
- **Amaranth**
- **Whole wheat or whole-grain bread** (check the label)
- **Whole wheat or other whole-grain pasta**
- **Whole wheat couscous**
- **Whole-grain crackers** (the kind that are minimally processed, with little or no fat)
- **Whole wheat and other whole-grain flours**

FLEXIBLE FRUITS AND VEGETABLES

Though still very nutritious, a few fruits and vegetables are Flexible because they're more calorie dense than other fruits and vegetables. The list is short:

- **Avocados**
- **Corn**
- **Peas**
- **Potatoes** (all kinds)
- **Coconut**
- **Tropical tubers** (like yucca, cassava, and taro)
- **100 percent fruit and vegetable juices**

NUTS AND SEEDS

Nuts and seeds are excellent sources of protein, unsaturated fat, vitamins, fiber, and other nutrients. Their crunch makes them ideal for snacking and—as you know—ground to a butter, they're a favorite. (Apple with almond butter—nothing better.) But their relatively high calorie density throws them into the Flexible Foods category. And, like potato chips, they can be hard to stop eating once you get started, so try to take just a handful, and always eat them with fruit or other foods in the Unlimited Foods camp. (You can also slow down by cracking your own.) Seek out the most natural form of nuts—raw or roasted, with salt if you like—but stay away from any coated in oil or sugar, like cayenne-honey-glazed pecans. You still have lots of options:

- **Almonds**
- **Peanuts** (technically a legume)
- **Cashews**
- **Hazelnuts** (filberts)
- **Pecans**
- **Pistachios**
- **Macadamia nuts**
- **Walnuts**
- **Pumpkin seeds**
- **Sesame seeds**
- **Poppy seeds**
- **Flax and chia seeds**

OILS

Choose minimally processed, flavorful, unsaturated fats. There's more about all these on pages 132–133, but always avoid hydrogenated fats like vegetable shortening; and don't rely on vegetable-based saturated fats like coconut and palm oils. The best are these:

- **Olive oil**
- **Sesame oil**
- **Sunflower, grapeseed, peanut, or other vegetable oils**
- **Nut oils**

SWEET CONDIMENTS AND SWEETENERS

This is an odd list, with many seemingly incongruous items; what they have in common is sugar. (If you do buy them, try to find versions that don't contain high fructose corn syrup.) Many packaged condiments are surprisingly high in sugar; even salad dressings can be packed with added sugar and chemicals, which is why I urge you to make your own (see page 232). Many of these condiments break the five-ingredient rule (see page 76), but you don't use much, and they add flavors that—because of their familiarity—can help you make the transition from the SAD.

- **Oat milk**
- **Rice milk**
- **Nut milks** (almond and hazelnut are most common)
- **Soy milk**
- **Barbecue sauce**
- **Ketchup**
- **A-1 Sauce**
- **Relishes and chow-chows**
- **Sweet pickles**
- **Maple syrup** (grade B packs the most punch and is cheaper than grade A)
- **Honey** (not technically vegan)
- **Sugar** (turbinado is the least processed)

TREATS

At last, the after-6 P.M. foods. I wouldn't dream of cutting these items out of my diet, but I don't eat them nearly as often—or in as large quantities—as I used to. Yes, you can eat Treats during the day if you are careful to balance out the rest of the day—or series of days, or week—by being more strict. For VB6 beginners, though, that kind of flexibility can be like quicksand; better to stick to the plan until you get the hang of it. And there's no reason not to: Look at all the goodies you can eat every evening:

MEAT

As outlined on pages 73–75, VB6 encourages you to think about using meat as a garnish rather than a centerpiece. (And if you're worried about getting enough protein, don't be: Reread pages 59–62, and also check out the nutrition information that follows the recipes.) All meats are in the Treats category, including any others not on this list:

- **Chicken**
- **Beef**
- **Pork**
- **Turkey**
- **Eggs** (and products made with eggs, like custard and mayo)

- **Lamb**
- **Smoked and cured meats** (like bacon, sausages, salamis, hams, and so on)
- **Venison and other game meats**
- **Duck, goose, pheasant, quail, and other bird**

DAIRY

Though VB6 views all dairy as a treat, some is better than others. Instead of processed cheese and sugary flavored yogurt, look for real milk and cream, plain cultured yogurt, and well-made, flavorful cheeses. For more suggestions about how to shop for dairy, see The VB6 Pantry starting on page 129. But in general, gravitate toward those listed below, and eat them only after 6 o'clock:

- **Hard cheeses:** Parmesan, Cheddar, manchego, other aged and dried cheeses
- **Soft cheeses:** Aged mozzarella, feta, Monterey jack, Muenster, blue cheeses, Brie
- **Fresh cheeses:** Fresh mozzarella, ricotta, mascarpone, fresh goat cheeses, quark

- **Milk**
- **Butter Cream**
- **Sour cream**
- **Yogurt** (preferably plain; the fat content doesn't matter)
- **Buttermilk**
- **Crème fraîche**

FISH AND SEAFOOD

Fish and seafood are the healthiest animal proteins you can eat, in large part because they have less saturated and more beneficial fats than other animal products. But despite fish's undeniable health benefits, the disastrous and unsustainable state of fishing practices makes it difficult to recommend eating it very frequently. (There are also contamination problems, and very real problems with aquaculture, or fish farming.) Add to that the challenges of being able to correctly identify sustainable species, and it becomes a tricky business. So it's difficult to recommend fish as a daily food, even though in general it's better for you than meat. (To keep track of what's best check the listings at www .montereybayaquarium.org/cr/seafoodwatch.aspx.) In any case, here's how you can look at fish to help you make good choices and substitutions in recipes:

- **Thick fish fillets:** Salmon, cod, hake, halibut, bass, char, striped bass, etc.
- **Thin fish fillets:** Mackerel, flounder, trout, tilapia (which I don't really fancy much for its flavor or texture), catfish
- **Fish steaks:** Salmon (wild is best), swordfish, halibut
- **Small-to-medium whole fish:** Anchovies, sardines, smelt, whiting, porgies, mackerel
- **Shellfish and mollusks:** Shrimp, clams, mussels, oysters, lobster, crab, crawfish, langoustines, squid, octopus

"THE WHITE STUFF," OR PROCESSED CARBS

When a food goes from brown to white, it's a signal something has been removed—usually most or even all of the good stuff. Hyper-processing reduces nutrition, and *really* reduces fiber. (See page 36 for an eye-opening comparison.) Make no mistake: I can't live without white pasta, rice, or bread. But I no longer eat these things throughout the day, or even daily. That's why "white stuff" is considered a Treat:

- **White pasta**
- **White rice**
- **Good white breads:** The crusty, airy kind from a good baker (including yourself) is too satisfying and delicious to pass up sometimes.
- **Egg breads:** Challah, brioche, and the like.
- **Sandwich breads, pizza, or focaccia**
- **White flour:** For breading and other baking.
- **Crackers:** Regardless of what they're made of—gluten free, whole grain, or otherwise—they're still processed and they're still treats.

ALCOHOL

Well, talk about empty calories: Nothing is emptier than alcohol, or more controversial. There are carbohydrates in alcohol, and they're digested fast, like sugars; from a strictly dietary point of view, alcohol is no better than white bread, just a tiny step above soda. And, of course, there are people who have problems with alcohol that go way beyond diet. But if you're not one of those, and you drink moderately, there's evidence that alcohol is physically good for you. And, of course, it can help you relax. More than anything else in the VB6 diet, alcohol is a judgment call: definitely off limits during the day, and up to you at night. But if you're seriously trying to lose weight, very limited drinking—or none at all—is something you should consider.

DESSERT

Dessert, of course, is the quintessential treat. There's always a special moment when you take your first bite, and that's the feeling you want to capture whenever you reach for something sweet. No one's saying you have to give up desserts and sweets, but you do need to learn to savor and limit your indulgences: A small piece of cake is almost always just as good as a big one. I know this is easier said than done, but *practice*— the rewards make it worth it. And try eating some fruit for dessert before you reach for the baked goods or candy.

I'm not including dessert recipes in this book; I don't like fake desserts and I don't do them, and you probably have plenty of recipes for real ones already. My only suggestion is that you choose good-quality, preferably homemade, sweet treats—or a piece of dark chocolate or caramel—over a bag of supermarket cookies. The difference in satisfaction will be huge, and you'll be avoiding ingredients you don't know or want. And if you're at all like me, you'll find that after a week or so eating VB6, your cravings for sugar will be sharply diminished.

HYPER-PROCESSED AND JUNK FOODS

A certain amount of judgment is required here, because this category represents a full spectrum: Imported pasta from Italy is undeniably a processed food, but in terms of its number of recognizable ingredients, it's a far cry from a doughnut. Still, I promised that VB6 wouldn't forbid any foods, and it won't. But I hope by now you recognize the importance of limiting—drastically—the sorts of foods on this list:

- **Fast food:** Yes, there are some chains and local restaurants that offer decent choices, but you have to be selective and resist temptation.

- **Protein, granola, or so-called diet bars:** Just eat real candy; it will feel more like dessert, is likely to contain more real food, and might even have fewer calories.

- **Frozen meals:** Yes, even "diet" ones. Besides, in the time it takes to heat one up, you could cook something.

- **Chips:** All kinds, fried, baked, or otherwise.

- **Packaged salty snacks:** Especially the super-salty powdery snacks like Doritos, Cheetos, and Pringles.

- **Soda or sweetened beverages:** Including Gatorade, energy drinks, and sweet tea. (There's evidence that diet drinks aren't that good for you, either. Drink water.)

- **Packaged desserts:** Twinkies, doughnuts, packaged cookies, fruit roll-ups.

- **Sugary cereal:** Most packaged cereal, really. Even so-called healthy options and granola are filled with sugar.

PERSONALIZING YOUR APPROACH TO VB6

Okay: You know *what* you'll eat. Now let's talk about *how* you'll eat. Once you're familiar with the three VB6 food groups, it's easy to make up your own meal plans, whether you're cooking at home or eating out, or to make substitutions to the plan described on page 119.

But first, consider this question: What kind of eater are you?

Let's state the obvious: No two people are alike, yet most weight-loss plans assume that the same approach will work for everyone. No allowances are made for your current eating habits, your behavioral patterns—who you are or what you like to eat. To be both effective and sustainable, a diet must acknowledge that each of us has our own quirks, tastes, cravings, interests, and living situations that affect our food choices. And no diet will succeed unless it can accommodate these differences.

To help figure out how VB6 can work best for *you*, I've identified six broad categories, each representing a different eating style, with suggested specific tips and tools for each to help tailor VB6 to that style. You may find that, like me, you're a mix of two or more kinds of eaters. I'm an avid runner, so in one way I fall into the Athlete category (at least some weeks!)—yet my professional life puts me squarely in both The Cook and The Restaurant Regular boxes as well. And since I have always cooked meals for my family, even though my daughters are grown I know what it's like to have young ones in the house. I don't rely on the mainstays of the SAD, though I do resort to fast food at times when I'm on the road. And since I've been doing VB6, I've become more of The Grazer, nibbling and snacking my way through the day.

The main point here is self-evaluation, but a practical one: The more honest you are, the better. Remember: We're working toward a lifetime of good eating and good health. Some of you will start on this path literally playing by the book: You'll turn to the 28-Day Plan on page 119 and dig in. Others will try the plan and tweak it as you go. Many of you will absorb the principles and the thinking behind the food groups and forge your own plan.

All three approaches—and anything in between—are utterly valid. And it doesn't matter how many of these categories you find yourself in; just use whatever tips will be helpful depending on what the day at hand brings. Take what you learn from these eater profiles and apply it it throughout the book to develop the tools you need to succeed.

THE ALL-AMERICAN

Like most people, you're time-crunched. Maybe you cook at home and maybe you don't, but in any case your diet is high in animal products and processed carbohydrates and relatively low in fruits and vegetables, whole grains, and beans. You drink soda and beer or wine instead of water. You frequently rely on packaged foods from the supermarket, often order takeout or fast food, or eat at restaurants.

YOUR ADVANTAGES
You're not alone—most of your friends and family are probably in the same boat. You realize you need to change your eating habits and maybe even those of others you care about.

YOUR CHALLENGES
Eating VB6 will involve breaking yourself free of the SAD. To make changes long term, your adjustments should be comfortable, whether that means gradual, drastic, or somewhere in between. Only you know which will work best for you, but the list that follows includes suggestions for both fast and slow approaches so you can try either—or both.

YOUR STRATEGY
• Reconsider "convenience." It often takes longer to order and receive your takeout delivery than it does to make a bowl of pasta or a stir-fry, especially if your pantry is well stocked.

• Set aside at least 20 minutes for eating each meal, then build to 30 minutes. Relax and enjoy.

• Choose cooking at home over eating out as often as possible. Make and pack lunch as often as you can.

• Gradually restock your pantry, getting rid of prepared food and replacing it with the items listed on page 129.

- Drink water instead of soda. Or unsweetened tea or coffee, or even diet pop if you must. But put down that poison.

- Include a vegetable dish or salad with every meal, or eat some fruit before or after. Put a fruit bowl on your counter and keep it full. Invest in a salad spinner.

- Try some of the snacks on page 182; you'll want to try more.

- Cook: Try some of the Restaurant Regular strategies on page 108. Look for VB6 recipes that are familiar and give them a whirl. Then move on to some of the less familiar alternatives.

- Make healthy eating a priority in your household budget. Get over the (wrong) notion that eating junk is cheaper than eating well. Don't let coupons dictate your shopping list.

- If you must get fast food, avoid eating in the car. Sit in the restaurant or bring the food home and eat it off of a real plate, not a wrapper.

- When you get discouraged or backtrack, skim through Part One to remind yourself of how far you've come, and how enormous the upside of changing your diet is.

TO ADJUST THE 28-DAY MEAL PLAN

If you're going for a big change quickly, use the menus to make weekly shopping lists and cooking schedules, adjusting each recipe to include the variations and ingredients that sound most appealing. For a more gradual approach, choose just one meal a day you're going to replace, and stick with that for four weeks. Then repeat the four-week plan, replacing additional meals with VB6 recipes until you're eating as many VB6-style meals and snacks as you can.

THE FAMILY GAL (OR GUY)

You've got other mouths to feed besides your own, and their needs or preferences may come first. You usually cook at home—a lot of chicken, simply cooked meat, cheesy casseroles, simple vegetables and salads. There are usually potatoes, bread, or noodles on the table, but meat is always the centerpiece of the meal.

You're already cooking, which is great. This means you have the power to change the way your family and loved ones eat, while helping everyone around the table eat better.

YOUR CHALLENGES

Your people need to eat, and they won't eat what they don't like, so you can't rock their world so hard that they mutiny and boycott dinner. Making changes to your routine might involve a little bit of extra work, but only at the beginning of the transition to VB6.

YOUR STRATEGY

• Put one familiar, beloved dish on the table every night, then surround it with a lot of VB6-friendly foods—like mashed sweet potatoes, sautéed spinach, *and* sliced tomatoes.

• Use your time in the kitchen efficiently to prepare salads and vegetables—in bulk, in advance—for future meals. See "Building Blocks," starting on page 228, for specific tips.

• When you cook vegetables, whole grains, or bean dishes make sure to prepare enough for leftovers.

• Deconstruct dinners: Instead of one-pot meals serve separate vegetable, starch, and (small-ish) meat dishes and let everyone balance his or her plate as desired, with you setting the example for a vegetable-driven diet. Reduce the amount of meat you serve and increase the amounts of everything else on the table.

• Evaluate your cooking techniques: Are you pan-frying when you could be roasting or broiling? Do you take advantage of the microwave for steaming fresh vegetables? How often do you make soup? Would using a slow-cooker be of help?

• Focus on ingredient swaps: Olive oil instead of butter, brown rice for white, whole wheat pasta for plain noodles.

• If you live in a house full of sugary cereal eaters, wean them by cutting their usual favorites with more nutritious whole-grain options. Or better still, make homemade cold or hot cereal (see pages 138 and 143).

- Pack lunches for everyone in the family. Make sure the kids get fruit and vegetables, even if you have to pack a sandwich with meat. (Though discourage that, too.) Adults get big salads or VB6-style leftovers.

- If you use treats as a reward, make sure they're healthy treats—at least half the time for starters.

- Make (or buy) a great dessert once or twice a week. The other nights, have plenty of cut fruit available and if there's a revolt, serve it with honeyed yogurt, a cookie, or a small scoop of ice cream.

- Put all willing and able bodies to work, helping you cook and clean up. It's a great way to bond, foster good habits, and lighten the load. Let your helpers decide which vegetables go into the stir-fry or soup.

TO ADJUST THE 28-DAY MEAL PLAN

Make VB6 family dinners the goal (at least for the beginning), making some adjustments or augmenting the menu with other dishes as described above. Then make yourself (and anyone who's game) the breakfasts and lunches, recognizing that you might be the only one eating vegan meals during the day.

THE RESTAURANT REGULAR

You love good food, but don't love to cook. Instead you—and everyone who shares meals with you, whether family or friends—almost always eat in restaurants, grab takeout, order in, or go to dinner parties. You appreciate good ingredients and consider yourself a little adventurous, even a "foodie." Perhaps your job requires you dine out or travel a lot. (That means you're in a lot of airports.) You strive to make healthy choices, but in the end you go for whatever sounds the most exciting at the time—and that's all catching up to you and your waistline.

YOUR ADVANTAGES

Eating is a pleasure you don't have to abandon with VB6. You'll only be adjusting proportions, increasing plant-based foods while the meat, dairy, desserts, and other foods decrease. Since you're deferring—and redefining—pleasure, you can still enjoy all the social and aesthetic aspects of eating in restaurants.

You need to spend at least a little time in the kitchen. And through this process, you will also learn how to make better choices—that is, have more discipline—when you do eat out.

YOUR STRATEGY

• Buy essential cookware and stock up on VB6-friendly foods as needed. (Page 94 is the place to start.)

• Dedicate some time—an hour a day would be fantastic—to cooking. Right now, nothing is more important. You may need to juggle your priorities, but you may be surprised at how easy it is to find some time.

• Remember: You don't need to become a chef. Just learn to cook a bit. If you can read a recipe, you can cook.

• Vary ingredients and seasonings to please your tastes. This will instantly elevate your cooking; what you produce in your own kitchen will taste as good as (eventually better than) the restaurant meals you're used to, because they will showcase the foods and flavorings you love most.

• Prepare breakfast at home, even if it's just hot cereal or whole-grain toast and fruit. Take it out the door with you if you must.

• Try making your favorite restaurant and takeout dishes the VB6 way by simply increasing the ratio of vegetables to meat, poultry, fish, or dairy and substituting whole grains and beans for animal foods wherever possible.

• Think of ways to make cooking fun and exciting: Play music, watch television, chat with friends, or enjoy the solitude.

• In restaurants, start your meal with vegetable soup, or make it your main course. (It's almost always the most VB6-friendly thing on the menu.) Get salad or fruit instead of fries or chips.

- Build lunch around a vegan salad. I frequently order a green salad and a couple of vegetable side dishes. Again, vegetable soup!

- Compose your restaurant meals creatively to break out of the meat main-dish mind-set: Order all side dishes or focus on vegetable-heavy appetizers and soups. Don't be apologetic about ordering what you want from the menu.

- If you're eating a special lunch out and want to enjoy animal foods, of course you can. But opt for a vegan dinner that night.

- Bring leftovers home. Brown rice from Chinese restaurants is a shortcut to another meal tomorrow.

- At dinner buffets and parties, start with salad and soup, then go back for non-vegan items if you're still hungry.

- When you grab takeout, choose simple components over multiple-ingredient dishes. Shop at supermarkets that have VB6-friendly prepared foods and takeout options. Take advantage of good-quality salad bars to stock your fridge with already-prepared food.

- If you drink alcohol daily, think about all the empty calories you're getting.

TO ADJUST THE 28-DAY MEAL PLAN

Use it mostly for structure. Pick out what you think you'd like to make at home and do as much cooking from the "Building Blocks" recipes as possible. Fill in with restaurant meals, using the dishes on the plan as the model for what dinner might look like.

THE COOK

You cook. You spend time each day planning meals and menus. You make choices based on the taste, color, texture, sometimes even the provenance, of ingredients. Your fridge and pantry are full, and you've always got a shopping list in the works. You spend a relatively large part of your income on food. You like to entertain and are frequently the guest of other good cooks. You probably eat out a fair amount, too, but only at restaurants where the food is as good as that you make yourself.

YOUR ADVANTAGES

You enjoy cooking, and that's a huge head start. Once you set your mind to it, you'll easily rebalance your diet into the VB6 way of eating.

YOUR CHALLENGES

You eat so well, it's hard to maintain—or lose—weight. Diets require you to give up too much, and a life of deprivation is just not worth it.

YOUR STRATEGY

• Unleash all of your cooking skills on VB6-style recipes, bringing what you know about varying ingredients and seasonings into the realm of plant-based dishes.

• Make more room in your fridge for fruits and vegetables. Cook key VB6 components like beans and grains; prepare fruits and vegetables. (You should be living in the "Building Blocks" chapter that starts on page 228.) Convert the deli drawer to a place for storing grains and beans of all types. And try at least one new type of grain *and* bean every week.

• Adjust your favorite recipes to be VB6 friendly. Turn your ratio of processed food and meat to vegetables upside down by doubling up on the vegetables and cutting the processed food or meat in half.

• Continue to make the foods you love but in smaller quantities. Don't make so much at dinner that you have meat-based dishes tempting you to eat them during the day. (This, I confess, is a problem I have all the time. Freeze or give away your meat-based leftovers; your co-workers will love you.)

• When you do cook larger quantities, cook animal foods separately from plant foods so you can store them separately and focus on the vegetables for next day's breakfast or lunch.

• Overshop in the produce section and at farmers' markets. You'll find a way to eat what you bring home, and if you don't, make soup to freeze for later. Whenever possible, replace butter with olive oil and minimize how much white flour, rice, and pasta you eat. (I repeat this for emphasis because I know how hard this is to do.) At most meals, replace the starch (or at dinner, the meat!) with another vegetable dish.

• Roast, broil, or grill instead of deep-frying or pan-frying whenever you can; you'll also likely be eliminating batters and breadings.

• Resist the urge to make fancy desserts more than occasionally. On other days, poach some fruit or enjoy a couple squares of good dark chocolate and a cup of fresh herb tea. Try dessert recipes that emphasize fruit and those where you can substitute whole grains or flours for some of the white flour.

• Use silken tofu as a thickener; try eating tofu, seitan, and tempeh; and if you like it, incorporate more into your repertoire.

• Halve the amount of cheese you would normally add to your dishes.

• Same caveat on booze as The Restaurant Regular: Be mindful of the empty calories you're getting from alcohol.

TO ADJUST THE 28-DAY MEAL PLAN
Follow the plan closely at first to get the hang of the plant-to-animal ratios then feel free to design your own menus in the VB6 mold.

THE GRAZER

You eat only when you're hungry and happily stop eating when you're full, and you eat small quantities throughout the day rather than sitting down for three big meals. (If you snack all day long *and then* eat three large meals, you're more of an All-American; see page 104.) You're less worried about the quantity of food you're eating than the quality of what's in your diet.

YOUR ADVANTAGES
VB6 might just easily have been called "The Grazing Diet," since you are welcome to eat as much of the unlimited foods as you like all day long. You'll be able to get more servings out of each recipe here, so you'll always have plenty for leftovers with minimal work.

You want to choose nourishing foods that keep you satisfied, and should plan ahead so that when you get hungry you always have Unlimited or Flexible Foods handy and don't reach for Treats.

YOUR STRATEGY

• Cook your own small meals and snacks at home as much as possible, using the VB6 recipes as a guide; they'll be more nutritionally balanced than most purchased snacks and you'll know what's in them. Invest in some airtight, portable containers in different sizes to portion out your snacks so you control the amount, as well as carry them easily with you wherever you go.

• Carry food with you and leave a good supply at your office, school, work, or wherever you spend a lot of time away from home.

• Avoid vending machines at all costs. Use vegetables and fruit as your go-to snacks. Eat nuts, too, but pack them in individual portions so you don't overeat them. (And choose raw, roasted or salted nuts, not sweetened or processed nuts.) When you get hungry, drink a glass of water before you snack.

• Avoid sugary—or other highly processed carbohydrate—snacks, which will just make you hungry again soon after eating.

• If you're out and are hungry, look for a supermarket or other place to buy VB6-friendly food; avoid convenience stores, vending machines, and fast-food restaurants.

TO ADJUST THE 28-DAY MEAL PLAN

Choose unlimited foods as your primary snacks; then if you're still hungry, add Flexible Foods. At mealtimes, save some of your food to eat a couple hours later.

THE ATHLETE

Regardless of your game or activity, exercise is a big part of your life. You may structure every day to fit in a workout, or you may work out whenever you get a chance, but you commit to a few times a week. You usually get hungry after workouts (or are hungry all day) and don't always make the best food choices.

YOUR ADVANTAGES

You probably exercise to improve or maintain your good health, so it's likely that you've already cultivated at least some good eating habits. Since you burn more calories than someone who leads a sedentary lifestyle, you can—and should—eat more.

YOUR CHALLENGES

Many exercisers actually put on weight or have a hard time taking it off because they find themselves hungry all the time; they might eat too much at mealtime or make poor snack and processed-food choices. Your goal is to eat so that you give your body enough calories to stay comfortable during and after activity, but not more than you need in order to lose or maintain weight—all the while developing an even healthier diet.

YOUR STRATEGY

- Avoid Gatorade and other "energy" or "sports" drinks. Plain water before, during, and after you exercise is fine.

- Eating VB6 provides plenty of protein, but if you want more, try increasing the amount of beans and whole grains in your diet before upping your dinnertime portions of animal protein. Tofu, beans, tempeh, and seitan are all concentrated plant-based sources of protein (see the sidebar on page 185).

- Choosing whole grains over processed carbohydrates will help you sustain your energy longer.

- Be sure to eat a hearty breakfast so you don't start the day behind in calories, which might cause you to overeat later. (I find it helps to eat at least a banana or a bowl of oatmeal before an early-morning workout.)

- Keep fruit and nuts with you always so you never let yourself get too hungry or weak.

- If you find you need more calories to fuel your workouts, increase your intake of Flexible Foods, not Treats. (See pages 96–99.)

- If you are exercising less (or more) than usual, adjust your food intake accordingly.

TO ADJUST THE 28-DAY MEAL PLAN

You can follow the plan closely if you'd like, changing individual recipes and serving sizes as described in the strategies above. And when you eat in restaurants or order takeout, layer the suggestions here onto the strategies for those profiles, too.

ENVISIONING A DAY OF VB6

Food is inseparable from life and your food is inseparable from you, as the preceding eater profiles demonstrated. To sustain the changes you're making, you must have confidence that you can integrate VB6 into your daily activities. So before outlining the 28-Day Plan, let's walk through some examples of what you might eat on a typical VB6 day, weaving in some examples of how some established VB6ers navigate the changes you'll be making.

BREAKFAST

If you usually drink juice in the morning, switch to a smoothie or have some fresh fruit. If you need caffeine, drink coffee, not cola or a sugary energy drink. Coffee itself can be tricky to convert to VB6 unless you take it black. At first, I cheated and put a splash of milk or half-and-half in my coffee. (Now I drink it black.) It's not a big cheat, but if lattes are your thing, try substituting unsweetened soy, oat, rice, or nut milk, since the amount of dairy that goes into even an average-size coffee drink is substantial.

Same goes with cereal: You're going to want nondairy milk, and you're going to want a decent cereal. Oatmeal with fruit is simple enough, and there's a basic whole-grain cereal recipe on page 138; there are also good store-bought options. Just make sure the sugar isn't sky-high and the ingredient list isn't Greek to you—the signal that the contents are highly processed.

I can eat—and enjoy—almost anything in the morning, including last night's leftover vegetables. I may eat beans or tofu, or drink a smoothie. I also try to have plain pre-cooked grains in the fridge, so all I have to do is pop them in the microwave. (There are lists of sweet and savory accompaniments on page 144.) A slice or two of good whole-grain toast is also a good option. Top with nut butter, hummus, or mashed beans if you want a little more heft. Otherwise, try mashing a little fruit with a fork and spreading it on your toast like jam.

In general, fruit is a good way to get the day rolling. Fruit salad feels more meal-like than eating an apple or banana out of hand, so think about cutting up fruit the night before while you're wrapping up in the kitchen. In an airtight container (maybe sprinkled with some fresh lemon juice), even bananas and apples won't get too brown. And it just makes life easier.

Most VB6 breakfast food is portable if you need to get out the door in a hurry. And if you find it tough getting to work (or wherever you go) on time, or just aren't hungry until later, it's easy enough to stock your desk or office kitchen with what you need so you can settle in and eat a little more leisurely.

On weekends, when there's time to do more cooking, I do. Sometimes I even have a couple of eggs (or bacon) in the morning. It's life, and there's no reason to let perfection be the enemy of good. The key of course is self-awareness and discipline—without guilt or beating yourself up. One way to make the diet work is to set the tone by remaining strictly vegan on weekend days and saving your eggs for evening; but you could also think of eggs as a treat for a week's work well done.

SNACKING

After a substantial breakfast, I can easily cruise all the way to lunch. If it was a bit more on the skimpy side, I'll grab more fruit and maybe more coffee midway through the morning to keep from becoming too hungry by lunchtime. Remember to drink lots of water in the morning, too, since most of us wake up dehydrated.

LUNCH

A VB6 lunch takes more planning, especially if you need to pack it up and bring it with you. This is where leftovers come in handy. With salad or vegetables already made (see the recipes on pages 231 and 233), you can pull together lunch on the fly. Sandwiches are always a good portable meal, as long as they're made right; see the sidebar on page 169 for vegan filling ideas.

It's relatively easy to figure out some combination of beans and vegetables for lunch, either by purchasing them from the salad or hot food bar or by bringing them from home. There are so many varieties and ways to cook beans, it doesn't feel like eating the same thing over and over, and they're pretty filling. I have come to really like tofu at lunch; I get that it's an acquired taste (the usual complaint, in fact, is that it has no taste), but prepared well, it's satisfying and flavorful. The recipes on pages 162 and 165 might make you a convert.

If you're in a restaurant, it's easy to find vegan options, especially if you order from the sides and salad sections of the menu. Soup is another good choice. And think about how many Middle Eastern, Indian, North African, and Asian restaurants are either purposefully vegan or just naturally lean that way.

If you had a serving of whole grains in the morning, you might skip them at lunch, especially if you're having other calorie-dense Flexible Foods at noontime or you know you're going to have plenty in the evening. (I also find that minimizing Flexible Foods and emphasizing Unlimited Foods for a couple of days can help me easily shed those extra few pounds I tend to pick up when I'm traveling.) Many VB6ers find that focusing on fruits and vegetables at lunch, in combination with a moderate serving of either grains or beans—but not both— helped them maximize weight loss.

When I have more time, I cook a more involved lunch, like one of the pasta or rice dishes on pages 203–208. Or I'll make a big batch of soup that I'll eat for lunch and have for the rest of the week. On other days I'm happy just to have a big salad or plate of vegetables. And you will be, too.

MORE SNACKING

Getting from lunch to dinner without a bite is almost always impossible for me. So I keep fruit handy in the afternoons, and usually rely on a handful or two of nuts to tide me over. Leftovers from lunch also help sometimes. Tea is nice, too, and strangely satisfying (it's clearly psychological but, hey, whatever works). If you're really hungry, have another serving of something from the Flexible Foods group (page 96).

DINNER

My work puts me in restaurants a couple of evenings a week. Since I'm eating after 6 o'clock, I eat whatever I want, and venture into Treat territory—but in moderation. The easiest way to avoid overdoing it is to order somewhat unorthodoxly: Instead of individual selections, get everything family style and pass things around. This way you can easily load up on the vegetable dishes and keep an eye on your meat portions. The same goes for dessert; sharing ensures you'll eat less and makes it easier to limit your intake to a couple of slowly enjoyed, satisfying bites.

When you're home and entertaining, follow the same model. You can cook far more salads and vegetables than fish, poultry, or meat; with the exception of soup, avoid plating food for your guests. If you're eating alone or with your significant other, keep dinner simple, like a bowl of pasta or a frittata and some salad. Some nights you'll probably find yourself skipping animal foods all together once you become comfortable eating VB6-style.

I—and anyone else I can hustle into volunteering—take advantage of every minute spent in the kitchen. So whether I'm cooking for myself and my wife or a crowd, I try to make enough extras for at least one lunch during the week. You can even make a future dinner easier by cooking roasts or stews in quantity and setting aside half. When I've got downtime between tasks, I almost always set a pot of beans or grains to boil or rinse and prep vegetables for snacking or salads later. (There's more about how to be efficient in the kitchen on page 228.)

Dinnertime can be an opportunity to share VB6 principles with those you care about most. I've always found that cooking with others can be incredibly rewarding, and everyone benefits by your good example. Continuing to eat lots of vegetables at dinner—as opposed to using the opportunity to chow down on SAD foods—will help keep you on track without making it feel like you're "on a diet." Whatever it is, getting support from others going through the same journey can be extremely comforting and give you strength, while challenging you to keep nurturing your new habits.

LATE NIGHT

No matter how good dinner was—or how rich the dessert—many people experience the time before bed as a gauntlet that sabotages the entire day. (I'm not usually tempted late at night because I eat fairly late and go to bed not long afterward, but I get it, especially when an early supper and kids are involved.) Here, frozen fruit can be the savior, especially berries, cherries, and peaches, which feel so luxurious. If you're game for a little more time in the kitchen, you can toss them into a food processor and make instant sorbet, a far more productive activity than sitting watching TV. A reasonable-size bowl of popcorn isn't a bad choice either. Another solution is to wait to have dessert—which might also simply be fruit, maybe with a little sweetened yogurt or some ice cream—until the dishes are done and you're relaxing before retiring. And remember, no matter what happens after 6 o'clock, tomorrow's another day.

5

The VB6 28-Day Plan

VB6 takes planning—and cooking. This versatile set of menus features all of the recipes in the book, taking advantage of variations and possible substitutions to keep home-cooked meals fresh and varied. Lunches and dinners include side dishes where appropriate.

You might be most comfortable following this super-structured four-week scheme fairly closely. In fact, by using the variations and substitutions suggested with many of the recipes, you could repeat this 28-Day Plan for a long time without getting bored. And you'd certainly spend some time cooking, which would immerse you in the principles and quickly demonstrate how easy it is to adapt dishes so they're VB6-style.

But I recognize that in real life, you're not going to be cooking every single meal for the next four weeks. That's why I've included Weekly Wildcards on page 120. They provide VB6 solutions for many of the occasions you'll encounter, both special and ordinary, from lunch with colleagues to potlucks.

Still another option: Just use the plan as a springboard to make some or all of your own choices. As long as you primarily eat vegan food before 6 o'clock, whatever works for you is just fine. My goal here is to offer a flexible and useful tool that teaches how to eat VB6 by example. It's not boot camp.

If you decide to follow the plan—and build in additional Unlimited and Flexible snacks as you need them—you'll get about 40 percent of your calories from mostly beneficial carbohydrates, 40 percent from healthy fat, and 20 percent from lean protein each week. If you're cooking for one or two, you'll have leftover meals. I didn't build many repeats into the plan—mostly because I want to provide fresh options every day—but feel free to replace leftovers for any of the meals listed here, provided you're careful about maintaining the VB6 principles.

I wish you great success, excellent health, and happy eating!

WEEKLY WILDCARDS

No one cooks every meal at home for a month and I don't mean to suggest that you should. Instead, look to the suggestions here whenever you need to swap out a meal for some other planned (or unplanned!) eating situation.

DINER BREAKFAST

Oatmeal and fruit: Nothing sexy, but always a solid bet.

Whole-grain toast: With peanut butter and banana.

Home fries: With sliced tomatoes or salsa on the side.

Omelet, without the eggs: If the joint has mushroom, pepper, or spinach fillings, that means you can have sautéed vegetables; potatoes or wheat toast optional.

Bacon and eggs: Well, of course, you can go for it—but either have a salad for dinner or consider this a non-VB6 day.

BRUNCH BUFFET OR DELI LUNCH

Salad table: Obvious, but start here and build. Load up on mostly greens and plain veggies to dress yourself; garnish with a taste or two of composed salad, which will probably provide enough dressing for your entire salad.

Omelet station: Ask the cook to sauté you up some vegetables, or get them raw for your salad.

Carving station: Avoid this station, or at least choose smoked fish. Either way, hit it last, after your plate is full, or even when you're done with your first plate; maybe you don't need it.

Dessert table: Stop at the fruit display first and put some colorful pieces on your plate. If you can't resist the sweets, share and keep portions small.

DELI LUNCH

Stir-fry: Always a good option, especially if it's all veggies.
Sandwich: A BLT, hold the bacon (add avocado), is a good idea.
Soup: Vegetable soup is almost always a perfect option.

FANCY LUNCH WITH THE BOSS

Salad: It's what she expects you'll get, so why not? If the menu only offers meaty options, get the house salad and soup or a couple of vegetable sides.
Soup: Get a bowl and build the meal around it.
Pasta: Hold the cheese and meat. Or not, and just re-think tonight's dinner.
A good piece of fish: This is a rare treat; make supper a soup.
Dessert: Yes, it's a shame to waste, but you might have to order it and not finish.

PIZZA PARTY

Hold the cheese: For lunch at least. You'll be surprised how good it is. Order one with a whole wheat crust if possible.
Side salad: If it's a good one, think about making this the meal.
Beer or wine: If it's a celebration, raise a glass.

SALAD BAR

Be thankful for all the vegan-ness.
Avoid the pitfalls (which you know).

CHINESE TAKE-OUT LUNCH

Soup: Unlikely any will be vegan (they're based on chicken stock), but egg drop, hot and sour, or greens-and-tofu are all better than wonton.
Egg roll: Have soup instead, or vegan fried (brown) rice.
Stir-fried Vegetables: Order something without the meat and ask for peanuts and/or tofu.
Steamed Vegetables: Better still. Drizzle them with dumpling dipping sauce, sesame chile oil, and rice vinegar or lemon.
Rice: Brown if they have it; white is no big deal once in a while. Or skip it all together.
Fortune cookie: Hopefully it comes with an orange; read the fortune, eat the orange.

(continued)

EVENING COCKTAIL PARTY

Crudités: Home base. Try dipping only every fifth piece or so.

Passed hors d'oeuvres: Let one platter of each go by before deciding what's best.

Meatballs: Can you stop at one? If not, veer toward the cocktail shrimp instead.

Cheese tray: There's fruit nearby, yes? Make this dessert.

Cocktails: If you want to drink, go ahead, but alternate each alcoholic glass with one of sparkling water.

FRIENDS' DINNER PARTY

Taste everything: But eat mostly vegetables.

DINNER OUT WITH FRIENDS (OR THE KIDS)

Family style: Pass plates to share and share alike. That way you can focus mostly on vegetables.

A la carte: You know what to do.

POTLUCK BARBECUE

Suit yourself: You can't count on anyone else to bring a great vegetable dish, so you'd better do it, and eat it first, before you get started on the meat dishes.

SIT-DOWN DINNER

Graciously served: No choice, so sit back and enjoy whatever you want to enjoy on your plate. Tomorrow's another day.

Advance order: Pick the entrée you want and eat only a reasonable amount of it, or ask for the vegetarian plate.

Bold moves: Explore other options—or simply more vegetables or an extra salad—with a friendly server.

WEDDING RECEPTION

Finger food: Make dinner of these or the main course; otherwise you may wind up eating two meals.

Do reconnaissance: Survey your options, then plan what you want to put on your plate.

Soup or salad first: Start with one or both; then see how it goes.

Cake: Of course; after your dinner has settled. Then get up and dance.

Champagne toast: Of course; then get up and dance some more.

Week 1	BREAKFAST	LUNCH	SNACK	DINNER
DAY 1	Homemade Cold Cereal with oat milk (page 138)	Eggplant Un-Parmesan (page 176) + Cooked escarole (page 233)	Frozen Banana Bonbons (page 195)	Crisp Celery Root and Chicken Cutlets (page 217) + Daily Salad Bowl (page 231)
DAY 2	Spiced Apple Jam and whole-grain toast (page 145)	Chickpea Ratatouille (page 167) + Daily Salad Bowl (page 231)	Spiked Guacamole (page 188)	Baked Ziti with celery, red onion, and pork (page 203) + Cooked spinach (page 233)
DAY 3	Breakfast Pilaf, Sweet or Savory, with brown rice (page 149)	Green salad with macerated pears and hazelnuts (page 158) + Top with cannellini beans (page 236)	Roasted eggplant spread (page 186) on carrots or whole-grain toast (page 142)	Sticks and Stones (page 219) + Brown rice (page 235)
DAY 4	Banana-tofu parfaits (page 140)	Lentil Salad (page 159) + Daily Salad Bowl (page 231)	Tortilla Crisps (page 192)	Braised Vegetables and Beef with mushrooms, carrots and onions (page 222) + Boiled new potatoes
DAY 5	Tex-Mex breakfast (page 154)	Easiest Vegetable Soup, with spinach and chickpeas (page 160)	Chocolaty Pineapple Kebabs (page 194)	Skillet Sweet Potatoes with Sliced Steak (page 220) + Daily Salad Bowl (page 231)
DAY 6	Scrambled Tofu with Spinach (page 155)	Black Bean Tacos with Tangy Cabbage (page 170) + Daily Salad Bowl (page 231)	Edamame (page 190)	Fisherman's Stew (page 211) + D.I.Y. breadsticks (page 243)
DAY 7	Corny Hoecakes (page 151)	One-Pot Pasta and Vegetables with fennel and tomatoes (page 172)	Vegan "Creamsicles" (page 193)	Zucchini Frittata, with or without Bacon (page 201) + Daily Salad Bowl (page 231)

Week 2	BREAKFAST	LUNCH	SNACK	DINNER
DAY 8	Fruity Nut Butter with whole-grain toast (page 141)	Baked Falafel with Tahini Sauce (page 180) + Daily Salad Bowl (page 231)	Crudités 24/7 (page 191)	Brown rice, risotto style, with mushrooms (page 207) + Cooked broccoli (page 233)
DAY 9	Hot Oatmeal (page 143)	Creamed Mushrooms on Toast (page 168)	Carrot Candy (page 184)	Steamed Vegetables and Seafood in Packages (page 213) + Daily Salad Bowl (page 231)
DAY 10	Blueberry Smoothie (page 139)	White bean salad (page 236) + Daily Salad Bowl (page 231)	Spiked Guacamole (page 188)	Meatballs, the New Way (page 224) + Tomato Sauce with Lots of Veggies (page 239) with whole wheat spaghetti
DAY 11	Fruity Nut Butter with steel-cut oatmeal (page 141)	Easiest creamy carrot soup (page 160) + Leftover white bean salad (page 236)	Kale chips Lacinato (page 184)	Succotash, Greens, and Sausage (page 225) + Daily Salad Bowl (page 231)
DAY 12	Tuscan breakfast (page 153)	Smashed and Loaded Sweet Potatoes (page 174) + Daily Salad Bowl (page 231)	Frozen Banana Bonbons (page 195)	Shrimp Tabbouleh (page 209) + Cooked kale (page 233)
DAY 13	Brown Rice Sweet Breakfast Pilaf (page 149)	Zucchini Un-Parmesan (page 177) + Daily Salad Bowl (page 231)	Tofu Jerky (page 189)	Hurry Curry with cauliflower, carrots, and peas (page 215) + Brown basmati rice (page 235)
DAY 14	Spiced tomato jam with whole-grain toast (page 145)	Now-or-Later Vegan Burgers (page 178) + Cooked carrots (page 233)	Roasted cauliflower spread (page 186)	Braised vegetables and chicken with fennel, and leeks (page 223) + Daily Salad Bowl (page 231)

Week 3	BREAKFAST	LUNCH	SNACK	DINNER
DAY 15	Banana Parfaits (page 140)	Greens and Beans Soup (page 164) + D.I.Y breadsticks (page 243)	Tortilla Crisps (page 192)	Steak and Broccoli Stir-fry (page 198) + Quinoa (page 235)
DAY 16	Homemade Cold Cereal with almond milk (page 138) + Broiled minty grapefruit (page 147)	Green Salad with macerated peaches and pecans (page 158) + D.I.Y. breadsticks (page 243)	Tofu Jerky (page 189)	Sticks and Stones (page 219) + Cooked cauliflower (page 233)
DAY 17	Turkish Breakfast (page 153)	Stewed Tomatoes and Beans (page 166) + Daily Salad Bowl (page 231)	Beet candy (page 184)	Cabbage, Sauerkraut, and Pork Chops (page 227) + Quinoa (page 235)
DAY 18	Scrambled Tofu with tomatoes (page 155)	One-Pot Asian Noodles and Vegetables with string beans and scallions (page 172)	Chocolaty Pineapple Kebabs (page 194)	Sweet potato frittata, with or without bacon (page 201) + Daily Salad Bowl (page 231)
DAY 19	Hot polenta (page 235) + Broiled Nutty Apples (page 146)	Creamed greens on toast (page 168)	Edamame out of the shell (page 190)	Meatballs, the New Way (page 224) + Daily Salad Bowl (page 231)
DAY 20	Tropical Toast (page 148)	Miso soup with spinach (page 162)	Vegan "Creamsicles" (page 193)	Baked Ziti with celery, carrots, leeks, and cheese (page 203)
DAY 21	Whole Wheat Hoecakes (page 151) with broiled nutty peaches (page 146)	Chickpea salad (page 236) + Cooked green beans (page 233)	Double green guacamole (page 188)	Fisherman's Stew (page 211) + Daily Salad Bowl (page 231)

Week 4	BREAKFAST	LUNCH	SNACK	DINNER
DAY 22	Spiced pear jam with whole-grain toast (page 145)	Portabella Un-Parmesan (page 176) + Daily Salad Bowl (page 231)	Crudités (page 191)	Steel-cut oats, risotto style, with asparagus (page 207) + Cooked spinach
DAY 23	Scrambled Tofu with bean sprouts (page 155)	Black Bean Tacos with Tangy Cabbage (page 170) + Cooked carrots (page 233)	"Vegan Creamsicles" (page 193)	Crab tabbouleh (page 209) + Daily Salad Bowl (page 231)
DAY 24	Hot quinoa (page 143)	Baked Falafel with Tahini Sauce (page 180) + Daily Salad Bowl (page 231)	Beet candy (page 184)	Crisp parsnip and Chicken Cutlets (page 217) + Cooked new potatoes
DAY 25	Fruity Nut Butter (page 141) with whole-grain toast	Vegetable miso soup with squash and tofu (page 162)	Spiked Guacamole (page 188)	Loaded Fried Rice with scallions, bell peppers, and snow peas (page 205)
DAY 26	Mango smoothie (page 139)	Now-or-Later Vegan Burgers (page 178) on top of Daily Salad Bowl (page 231)	Roasted cauliflower spread (page 186)	Braised Vegetables and Beef with celery root, leeks, and carrots (page 222) + Wheat berries
DAY 27	Hot-and-sweet breakfast pilaf made with quinoa (page 149)	Easiest red pepper and tomato soup (page 160) + Daily Salad Bowl (page 231)	Kale chips Lacinato (page 184)	Hurry Curry with Brussels sprouts, red peppers, and green beans (page 215) + D.I.Y crusty bread (page 243)
DAY 28	Turkish Breakfast (page 153)	Eggplant Un-Parmesan (page 176) + Polenta (page 235)	Kale chips Lacinato (page 184)	Steamed Vegetables and Seafood in Packages (page 213) + Daily Salad Bowl (page 231)

6

Cooking VB6

VB6, as I've promised, is about good food and real eating. You'll be able to eat real food, every day, for the rest of your life, and you'll never feel like you're on a diet. Whether you're a seasoned cook or a novice, my no-nonsense cooking advice and simple recipes will help you act on the plans described in Chapter 5—and change the way you eat forever.

All include variations and quick ideas, so you can cook from this book for months without eating the same thing twice. As you explore these recipes, you'll be learning to cook in a new way—a way that puts plants first, improves your health, and helps you lose weight.

ABOUT THE RECIPES

All the breakfasts, lunches, and dinners are one-dish meals, though you should feel free to add a salad, bread or grains, or more vegetables. (The plan starting on page 123 includes suggested sides to get you started.) Breakfasts and lunches are completely vegan; dinner dishes incorporate some meat, poultry, fish, eggs, or dairy. The snacks are just that: sweet or salty tidbits you can eat any time of the day when you might normally head for the vending machine.

"Building Blocks" recipes are make-ahead basics that will become the foundations of your everyday cooking: beans, whole grains, salad greens, and (real) dressings. Some take time, but none take much work or attention, and—especially if you make them in big batches—you'll use them. And that's the whole idea: They make cooking the VB6 way convenient, economical, and diverse.

Most recipes here make four servings, though there are some that serve six or eight. And that's the idea: Of course you can find packaged or frozen vegan food, and even take-out. But like the meat-based versions of "convenience" foods, they're usually loaded with chemicals and additives—which in my book still makes them junk.

A good part of the VB6 philosophy is that you will eat much better if you cook. Period. So, many of these recipes are designed to store and reheat well in the oven, toaster oven, or microwave; you can refrigerate leftovers for up to a few days, or freeze them for a few months. (The recipes and sidebars throughout this part of the book have lots of tips on exactly how to prepare and store extra food, and ways to reinvigorate the leftovers.) And if you freeze leftovers in individual servings, they're ready for a fast meal or snack at home or to bring to work, and they're just as convenient, giving you something to rely upon when you don't feel like cooking.

Because VB6 is not a point- or calorie-based diet, the serving sizes are just suggestions; you'll eat as much you want. (Consider the meal categories suggestions, too; you can eat dinner for breakfast, and vice versa; see Chapter 4.) But try starting with the recommended serving size (believe me: they're not small), enjoy your food, eat slowly, and pause before reaching for more. The recipes are also easy to multiply (or divide) so you can make larger (or smaller) quantities. This makes them useful for all occasions, from crazy weekday mornings to dinner parties or potlucks.

The estimated time it takes to make each recipe is also included; you'll find many in the 30-minute range. While some take more time, all are streamlined for speed—including clean-up. Try them; even if you're new to cooking, I'm confident you'll recognize that it can be as efficient as eating out, and has countless economic, health, aesthetic, and other advantages.

I've included nutritional information here largely because it's expected in diet books. Each profile (which was created using software that pulls from the USDA's nutrient database) reflects the first options from the recipe's ingredient list, identified specifically in cases where you have lots of choices. The impact variations and other suggested adjustments will have on the nutritional profiles depend on what substitutions you make: Generally, when you choose Unlimited foods, there won't be much change; Flexible foods will increase calorie counts by adding fat, protein, or carbohydrates.

You can ignore these numbers if you want—as I've said, you need not count *anything*, and I sure don't. (And as I've said, everyone processes calories and other nutrients differently.) So use these numbers—or those on labels for that matter—to inform yourself about what you're eating, but don't obsess about them.

THE VB6 PANTRY

All of this—cooking and eating well (and, really, *living*) is exponentially easier if your kitchen and pantry are up to speed. You don't need any special equipment: A basic collection of mixing bowls, pans, pots, baking sheets, knives, and simple tools like peelers and graters will cover it. If you have both room and budget, I recommend investing in a food processor and a blender. (If it has to be one or the other, go with the food processor.) I use both almost daily; the food processor streamlines chopping, slicing, and grating, and blenders make quick work of purees and smoothies.

The most important element of cooking my way is the VB6 pantry, which includes both perishable and long-storage ingredients. These foods are grouped according to the VB6 principles, beginning on page 94: Unlimited, Flexible, and Treats.

Don't feel like you have to buy everything on this list right away; many items are interchangeable with others in their group. (For instance, if you don't have quinoa, you can always substitute brown rice.) But aim to stock at least one ingredient from each group to start. As your repertoire and interests expand, you'll find new ingredients—grains, legumes, fruits, whatever—that will become favorites and you'll begin to substitute those you like best for those you like less. This is especially true with vegetables, where virtually everything in the same group is interchangeable. (See the lists starting on page 95 for examples.)

Generally, try to buy items from bulk bins so you can get as much or as little as you need. (And: Store grains, when you can, in the freezer or fridge; they'll keep much longer that way.) There are some packaged, canned, and jarred ingredients on this list, too; but always pay attention to the labels so you have some idea what you're getting.

Finally, the if-you've-got-it-you'll-eat-it theory works both ways: Keep junk within arm's reach and you'll likely grab it. Getting rid of that stuff makes eating it a nonissue. Many parents say they stock chips, cookies, microwaveable snacks, packaged pudding, and frozen pizzas for the kids, but then everyone ends up eating them. Instead of raising your kids on the SAD diet, think about getting them excited about the way you'll be eating, and allowing them to learn by the example you're setting.

End of lecture. On to the specifics:

THE UNLIMITED PANTRY

These start with aromatics, the staples that make everything else taste better (and are sometimes good on their own): onions, garlic, ginger, shallots, carrots, and celery, for example. Then there are vegetables that last for weeks in the fridge: most cabbages (including Brussels sprouts) and root vegetables. Sweet potatoes and winter squash are also keepers, best stored in a cool, dry, dark place like a cabinet—or in the fridge if there's room. Many other vegetables, like zucchini, radishes, broccoli, and cauliflower, will last a week in the fridge. Frozen vegetables complete the picture, and make prep a snap. (Some beans—like lima, fava, and black-eyed peas—are sold frozen, too.) And for fruit: All citrus lasts for weeks in the fridge, as do apples and pears. Buy more perishable items—like lettuce—as needed.

FRESH HERBS
All of these can make a huge difference in a dish, with little more effort than shopping and chopping. Parsley is the most useful—essential, I'd say—and versatile, especially in winter, but fresh mint, dill, rosemary,

oregano, chives, and thyme are really quite wonderful, and can be used somewhat interchangeably. (And some of these, most notably rosemary and thyme, will keep for weeks in the fridge.) Cilantro and basil are fragile, staying fresh for only a few days, but sometimes nothing else will do. For those tender herbs, rinse the entire bunch and put them in a vase or cup of water (like flowers) and refrigerate—they'll keep many days, often upward of a week, that way.

SPICES, CHILES, AND DRIED HERBS

Buy an assortment: They're inexpensive, don't need refrigeration, take up little room, and last for at least a year. My primary spices are cardamom, cumin, pimentón (smoked paprika), cinnamon, coriander, ginger, nutmeg, and fennel seeds. (You can buy these all pre-ground, or for even more flavor, toast and pulverize the seeds yourself in a coffee grinder.) Dried herbs are inferior to fresh but sometimes better than nothing (stick to sage, thyme, rosemary, oregano, and tarragon; don't bother with others). Stock whole dried hot and mild chiles, too; chipotles are great for their smoky heat. Spice blends, like curry and chili powders, are infinitely useful.

NON-SUGARY CONDIMENTS

Whole-grain and/or Dijon-style mustard is a must, as is vinegar. (I like sherry vinegar best; wine vinegars are also good, and balsamic is nice for drizzling on vegetables.) Horseradish (providing it doesn't contain cream, sugar, or other fillers) is handy for quick sauces. Also stock a good soy sauce (containing no more than soy, wheat, salt, water, and bacteria), and—if you don't make it yourself—good-quality jarred salsa. Hot sauces are optional.

CANNED TOMATOES

Convenient, inexpensive, and better than out-of-season "fresh." Whole plum (or Roma) tomatoes are sweetest and best-tasting, (crush them with your hands or work a knife through the can), but canned diced tomatoes are undeniably convenient. Steer clear of crushed or pureed tomatoes, which are watery, and avoid tomatoes with sugar added. Tomato paste is good, too: Choose tubes (like toothpaste) over cans, so you can use a bit at a time.

Sauerkraut. Pickles (without sugar). Roasted red peppers. Capers. Olives. These are all full-flavored ingredients with lots of uses, and they keep for months. Whenever possible choose glass containers over plastic and cans.

THE FLEXIBLE PANTRY

BROWN RICE AND WHOLE GRAINS

There are literally dozens of options here, and they're all interchangeable with some adjustments in cooking times. I like them all—from farro, kasha (toasted buckwheat), quinoa (one of my favorites), and millet to all kinds of brown rice, wild rice, steel-cut oats, and bulgur (partially cooked cracked wheat). Keep at least a couple of these around—again, store in the freezer or fridge for better keeping—and cook them in big batches.

BEANS

Beans come in hundreds of varieties. You can use canned beans in almost all of the recipes here but I cook my own—a big pot—90 percent of the time. There's no need to soak them first unless you happen to think of it ahead of time (they will just take a bit longer to become tender if cooked without soaking), and smaller beans, split peas, and lentils cook quickly. Then you can refrigerate or freeze them in small containers. This makes them as convenient as canned, *and* they're better and cheaper.

THE HANDFUL OF FLEXIBLE VEGETABLES

Potatoes, dried unsweetened coconut, tubers, and frozen peas and corn all keep well for at least weeks. Buy avocados rock hard and they'll ripen on the counter in a few days, without bruises.

OLIVE OIL

This should be your go-to fat. Extra virgin—which in theory at least means cold pressed and minimally processed—is what's important; don't worry too much about country of origin. I use the same oil for cooking and drizzling but of course you can buy one with more character for salads and drizzling if you want to splurge. Olive oil goes rancid quickly if it gets too warm or is exposed to light, so I buy big bottles (or cans), and keep only what I'll use in the next few days on the counter; the rest stays in its container in a cupboard or the fridge. (It clouds up and thickens when cold but returns to normal quickly at room temperature.)

OTHER OILS

When the flavor of olive oil isn't ideal—in Asian dishes, for example—or when you're cooking over high heat I call for "vegetable oil." There are a lot of choices under this umbrella, but some are better than others: Choose grapeseed, sunflower, safflower, or even peanut (it has a stronger taste that isn't as universal, but it's fantastic for stir-frying). Canola oil tastes bitter to me (and feels sticky), but it has a good nutritional profile so use it if you like it. As with olive oil, always look for minimally processed, high-quality oils, cold-pressed whenever possible.

NUTS AND SEEDS

As you like. Store in the fridge or freezer to prevent rancidity. I include unsweetened shredded coconut (which comes in both fine and longer strands) and nut butters in this category, too.

PASTAS AND NOODLES

Pasta made from white flour (which comprises all "regular" pasta) qualifies as a "treat," but the options for true whole-grain pasta—the kind that has no white flour in the ingredient list—seem to improve every year. There's pasta made from whole wheat, brown rice, farro, kamut pasta, and buckwheat. The best usually comes from Italy, although the best dried rice or soba (buckwheat) noodles are from Asia.

TOFU OR SILKEN TOFU

Firm tofu (usually packed in water) is chewy, and soaks up the flavor of whatever you cook it with. Silken or soft tofus packed the same way (but also available in airtight, shelf-stable boxes) are creamy and custard-like, and make a good stand-in for dairy in purees, soups, and dressing. All packaged tofu is usually dated, but if not, store refrigerated bricks of firm tofu in water in the fridge for up to a couple of weeks. Silken tofu in a box will keep in the cupboard for months; refrigerate it after opening.

COCONUT, ALMOND, OAT, SOY, OR OTHER NON-DAIRY MILK
Choose your favorite (I like oat milk in regular coffee, soy in cappucino), and use at will in place of cow's milk. So-called light or reduced-fat milks work just as well as full-fat kinds in most recipes. There's more about all of these in the sidebar on page 137.

BAKING INGREDIENTS
Even though there are limited baking (and no real dessert) recipes in this book, these are worth mentioning. Baking soda, baking powder, and instant yeast are requisite for most baking endeavors. Opt for whole wheat flour instead of all-purpose white whenever you can; you can use "white whole wheat flour" if you prefer (I don't). If you have gluten allergies, cornmeal, polenta, brown rice flour, or nut flours are excellent substitutes; use a packaged gluten-free baking blend in recipes that call for wheat flours without making other adjustments.

THE TREAT PANTRY

MEAT, EGGS, DAIRY, AND FISH
Since these are treats, I list only those that are long-keeping:

Parmesan cheese: Real Parmesan (Parmigiano-Reggiano) lasts for months in the fridge if tightly wrapped. (Grano Padano and many other dried Italian cheeses, like Pecorino Romano, are also good.) Always buy a hunk, not pre-ground stuff. Grated over any salad, vegetable, rice, or pasta dish, it provides flavor you can't get elsewhere.

Bacon: Keep a chunk (or some slices) in the freezer. A little goes a long way, especially in a stew, stir-fry, or pasta sauce. Same goes for guanciale, pancetta, speck, or any cured specialty meat.

Eggs: Still among the most versatile and nutritious of all animal products.

Butter: Even a tablespoon can round out a dish, and has no more fat or calories than vegetable oils.

Canned or jarred fish: Anchovies add huge amounts of flavor; sardines, salmon, and tuna are among the healthiest animal products you can eat.

"WHITE" FLOUR, PASTA, RICE, AND NOODLES

All keep for a long time, of course. White flour should be unbleached. For white rice, choose short grain or basmati (jasmine is really nice too). And, not surprisingly, the best pasta comes from Italy. (Rice noodles, made from rice flour, are good in many Asian noodle dishes.)

DRIED FRUIT

Raisins, cranberries, apricots, pineapple, dates, figs, and so on are delicious and convenient, but quite high in sugar; stick to fresh fruit whenever possible. Otherwise, keep portions small, and reserve these for special occasions or as flavorful additions to salads, bean dishes, pilafs, and desserts.

SWEETENERS

Whenever possible choose less refined alternatives to sugar—turbinado or "raw" sugar, maple syrup, agave nectar, or honey (which technically isn't vegan).

SWEETENED CONDIMENTS

Ketchups, relishes, and barbecue sauce—as well as fruit syrups; caramel, or sweet glazes or sauces—all contain a fair amount of sugar or other sweeteners. This doesn't mean you can't eat them (though some contain fewer undesired ingredients than others and in most cases you're better off making your own), but consider doing so a treat.

7
Breakfast Recipes

Dairy, eggs, and meat are all front and center in the SAD breakfast, which is often like diving into a sugar bowl, heavy with baked goods or sweet condiments like maple syrup or jams and jellies. Then there are breakfast meats. Not the best way to start the day.

But transitioning from the SAD toward a VB6-type breakfast isn't particularly difficult. At first I regularly craved a bagel with cream cheese or a pile of bacon. But my habits changed quickly—not instantly, but over the course of just a few weeks, so give yourself time—and now I enjoy my new morning rituals as much as I did the old ones.

For a while, steel-cut oats were a standby, though I often enjoyed other grains like wheat berries or brown rice, either with a drop of maple syrup or some soy sauce (and chopped celery—fantastic), or even nori. I reached for oat milk routinely and started to make smoothies with silken tofu.

As my habits changed, so did my cravings; the two fueled each other and bolstered my resolve. (It didn't hurt when I lost weight, either.) Now I look forward to whatever the morning might offer: stir-fried greens and tofu, polenta with oat milk, or some of last night's roasted vegetables with whole-grain bread. I always liked nontraditional breakfast foods, so all of this seemed like an opportunity to me.

But that's me. You might prefer to stick to one or two more familiar breakfasts—like oatmeal with fruit, a smoothie, or a fruit salad. And those are all great options.

MILK WITHOUT DAIRY

Given that many or even most people are lactose intolerant or allergic to milk, vegan milks are good regardless of VB6. They're made from oat, rice, soy, hemp, combinations of grains, and various nuts, and are now available everywhere, both in the refrigerator case and in shelf-stable packaging. Try different kinds until you settle on those you like best.

Choose an unflavored, unsweetened variety; they all contain a fair amount of natural sugar, usually in the form of glucose. (Cow's milk also contains a lot of natural sugar.) Unlike dairy milk, none of these contains residues of hormones or antibiotics, and many are made from organic grains. Some contain some kind of gum to keep them from separating (as if we couldn't shake the container!), and—like dairy products—they're sometimes enriched with vitamins.

You can even make your own vegan milk: Put 1 cup of dried unsweetened coconut, rolled oats, or nuts in a blender with 2 cups boiling water. Pulse the machine on and off to help prevent the hot liquid from spurting out the top. Then hold the top on tightly and let the blender run for at least 15 seconds. Let the mixture steep for 15 minutes; strain, preferably through cheesecloth, pressing on the solids to squeeze out as much milk as possible. Put the milk in a jar with a tight lid (discard the solids) and refrigerate.

HOMEMADE COLD CEREAL

MAKES: 8 SERVINGS   TIME: 15 MINUTES

So superior to store-bought you may never go back. Uncooked rolled oats—sweet, crunchy, and chewy—provide the base, and the rest of the mixture is totally customizable. Serve with fruit and you're set until lunchtime.

3½ cups rolled oats

½ cup mixed chopped nuts and seeds (like almonds, walnuts, pecans, cashews, sunflower seeds, or flax seeds)

½ cup raisins or other chopped dried fruit

¼ cup unsweetened grated coconut

½ teaspoon cinnamon or cardamom, or to taste

Pinch salt

4 cups soy or oat milk, or other nondairy milk, for serving

1   Combine the oats, nuts and seeds, raisins, coconut, and spices in a large bowl. Store in an airtight container in the fridge for up to 2 months.

2   To serve, put about 1 cup in a bowl and top with ½ cup milk. If you have time, let the bowl sit for 5 to 10 minutes to let the oats absorb some of the milk so they'll soften and sweeten.

NUTRITIONAL INFO *per 1 cup serving (made with almonds and served with soy milk):*
Calories: 288 • Cholesterol: 0mg • Fat: 12g • Saturated Fat: 5g • Protein: 10g • Carbohydrates: 38g • Sodium: 81mg • Fiber: 7g • Trans Fat: 0g • Sugars: 8g

FRUIT SMOOTHIE

MAKES: 4 SERVINGS   TIME: 5 MINUTES

A smoothie is one of the easiest and most satisfying ways to load up on fruit and its fiber while using whatever's lying around in your fridge or freezer. (You can even use vegetables; see the sidebar.) Coconut milk will make the richest smoothie, but even the "lite" versions have a fair amount of fat, so I cut it with a bit of fruit juice. Silken tofu (which is high in protein) becomes creamy and thick in the blender; it's great stuff, so please try that also. (For more about tofu, see page 133.) And don't worry about freezing the banana; if you forgot, just add a handful of ice to the blender instead of water.

3 cups unsweetened frozen or fresh fruit, any combination (strawberries, blueberries, peaches, mango, melon, etc.)

1 frozen banana

1 cup coconut milk, other nondairy milk, or silken tofu

½ cup unsweetened apple or orange juice, or more if needed

½ teaspoon vanilla, optional

Put all the ingredients in a blender and puree until smooth, adding a little water if necessary to get the machine started. Stop the machine to scrape down the sides once or twice. Serve immediately.

NUTRITIONAL INFO *(1¼ cup serving, made with mixed fruits, coconut milk, and unsweetened apple juice)*:
Calories: 240 • Cholesterol: 0mg • Fat: 13g • Saturated Fat: 11g • Protein: 3g • Carbohydrates: 32g • Sodium: 10mg • Fiber: 3g • Trans Fat: 0g • Sugars: 23g

BANANA PARFAITS

MAKES: 4 SERVINGS   TIME: 10 MINUTES

Mashed bananas give you all the creamy richness and sweetness you expect in a parfait without a bit of dairy. For an even creamier version, try the variation with silken tofu.

> 2 ripe medium bananas
>
> 2 tablespoons fresh lemon juice
>
> ½ cup low-sugar, high-fiber cereal (like the one on page 138)
>
> 3 cups berries or other chopped fresh fruit, or 1 cup Fruit Compote (page 230)

1. Put the bananas in a medium bowl and squeeze the lemon juice over all. Mash and stir the mixture with a fork or potato masher until it's as smooth or lumpy as you like.

2. Assemble parfaits in short, wide glasses in alternating layers of mashed banana, cereal, and fruit until you use everything up. Serve immediately.

BANANA-TOFU PARFAITS For a little more protein, substitute 1 cup silken tofu for one of the bananas. Proceed as above.

NUTRITIONAL INFO *(made with 2 tablespoons Homemade Cold Cereal, page 138)*: Calories: 198 • Cholesterol: 0mg • Fat: 3g • Saturated Fat: 1g • Protein: 3g • Carbohydrates: 41g • Sodium: 11mg • Fiber: 6g • Trans Fat: 0g • Sugars: 21g

---

D.I.Y. VEGETABLE AND FRUIT JUICE

You don't even need a juicer: All it takes is fresh fruit and/or vegetables, water, and a blender. Trim and seed the fruits and vegetables as needed, cut them up a bit, and put everything in the blender with enough water to get the machine going. (Some grated ginger can be really nice, too.) Blend until very smooth, adding more water or ice to thin or chill as you like.

You can drink the juice as is, or pass it through a mesh strainer (you'll be filtering out its fiber, though). The result will be fresher and more nutritious than bottled juices, faster than waiting in line at a juice bar, and *way* cheaper than either.

FRUITY NUT BUTTER

MAKES: 4 SERVINGS   TIME: 5 MINUTES

To make nut butter at home, all you do is put a bunch of nuts in the food processor with a few drops of water and let the machine work its magic; in a few minutes, you're done. Using fruit instead of water makes the nuts even better, reducing the spread's calorie density and adding bright freshness, color, and flavor, giving you a kind of instant pb&j.

You don't have to eat this on bread; try it on plain cooked grains or apple slices, or scooped up with carrot, celery, or jícama sticks.

    1 cup almonds or other nuts (see below)

    2 cups chopped fresh or thawed frozen peaches

    1 tablespoon fresh lemon juice

Put the nuts in a food processor and grind to a course meal. Add the peaches and lemon juice, and process, stopping as necessary to scrape down the sides of the bowl, until thick, creamy, and smooth, 3 to 4 minutes. Use right away, or refrigerate in a sealed container for up to 3 days.

NUTRITIONAL INFO *(for about ⅔ cup made with almonds and peaches):*
Calories: 241 • Cholesterol: 0mg • Fat: 18g • Saturated Fat: 1g • Protein: 8g • Carbohydrates: 16g • Sodium: 0mg • Fiber: 6g • Trans Fat: 0g • Sugars: 9g

---

SUBSTITUTIONS

Other fruit and nut combinations work just as well:

Apple and walnut	Strawberry and	Mango and cashew
Pear and pecan	pine nut	Blueberry and
Apricot and	Banana and peanut	macadamia nut
pistachio		

THE BEAUTY OF FROZEN FRUIT

No one can argue with a juicy summer peach or a crisp fall apple, but there are few things more disappointing than tasteless, mealy, out-of-season fruit. Frozen fruit is a terrific alternative. Not only is it fairly cheap and convenient, but since it's frozen at its peak, the color, flavor, and nutritional quality are often superior to those of out-of-season fresh fruit. (I always keep a few bags of frozen fruit stashed away in the freezer for this recipe, and for those on pages 139 and 140).

TOAST TALK

Whole grains are near-ideal morning food, but when you can't get it together to cook up a batch, whole-grain bread is a fast alternative. It will help you get out of the house well fed, especially if you're weaning yourself from bagels and cream cheese.

Look for true whole-grain bread, flatbread, or crackers. Whole wheat is always a better option than white, but remember that something can legally be sold as whole wheat as long as it contains *some* whole wheat flour. You've got to read the labels to find bread made from only whole grains. (100 percent rye is most common.)

Slice per slice, whole-grain loaves are higher in calories than white bread—which literally has been stripped of fiber, protein, and nutrients—but with those calories come loads more healthy protein and fiber that will keep you satisfied longer.

Some ideas for morning toast: Fruity Nut Butter (page 141), Spiced Apple Jam (page 145), or Fruit Compote (see page 230). To go savory, try a Turkish Breakfast (page 153) or top with Scrambled Tofu with Spinach (see page 155). Toast can also be a terrific vehicle for leftovers, loaded up with veggies from yesterday's meal, drizzled with olive oil or soy sauce or seasoned any way you like.

HOT OATMEAL (AND MANY OTHER CEREALS)

MAKES: 4 SERVINGS   TIME: 15 MINUTES, OR MORE DEPENDING ON THE GRAIN

Oatmeal is probably the first thing that comes to mind when you think of hot cereal, but other grains make delicious porridge, too. And you can take them in whatever direction you like—sweet, or savory, or both. (See the sidebars that follow.) Keep in mind that some suggestions are Unlimited Foods and others aren't.

This recipe makes four servings, and I encourage you to double it. The leftovers store perfectly in the fridge or freezer. You can divide the cereal into individual portions to reheat in the microwave or a small saucepan over medium-low heat. That way, a from-scratch hot breakfast becomes as fast as "instant."

> 2 cups rolled oats
>
> 1 teaspoon salt, plus more to taste

1 Stir together the oats, salt, and 4 to 4½ cups water (more water makes for creamier cereal) in a medium saucepan. Bring to a boil over high heat, lower the heat so the mixture bubbles gently, and cook, stirring frequently, until the water is just absorbed, about 5 minutes. Add water if necessary to keep the cereal from sticking.

2 When the grains are soft and the mixture is thick, taste and add more salt if you'd like. Serve with one (or a few) of the additions from the list in the sidebar. Store extra servings, covered, in the refrigerator for up to a week or in the freezer for up to 2 months.

NUTRITIONAL INFO *(1¼ cup oatmeal topped with 1 cup fresh strawberries):*
Calories: 323 • Cholesterol: 0mg • Fat: 6g • Saturated Fat: 1g • Protein: 14g • Carbohydrates: 57g • Sodium: 244mg • Fiber: 9g • Trans Fat: 0g • Sugars: 3g

---

OTHER GRAINS TO COOK THIS WAY

Use the method in the main recipe to cook any of the grains below. The cooking time will vary from 10 to 30 minutes, depending on the grain. So until you become familiar with them, check them often while stirring. They're listed in order of shortest to longest down each column:

Rolled rye or barley	Cornmeal	Quinoa
Rolled wheat	Cracked wheat	Millet

STIR-INS AND TOPPINGS FOR HOT CEREAL

SWEET

Chopped fresh fruit

Fruit Compote
(page 230)

Chopped dried fruit

Chopped nuts or
seeds

Maple syrup or
agave nectar

Nondairy milk

Unsweetened
grated coconut

Chopped dark
chocolate

SAVORY

Chopped cooked
vegetables

Chopped or grated
raw vegetables

Chopped fresh
herbs or scallions

Minced fresh or
crumbled dried
chiles

Fresh, cooked, or
bottled salsa

Grated ginger

Soy sauce

Olive oil

Sesame oil

MAKE-AHEAD BREAKFASTS

It's a cliché, but for good reason: Skipping breakfast—the most primitive and probably most common weight loss "strategy"—can throw your metabolism out of whack for the entire day, prompting you to overeat at lunch, and possibly even dinner and into the night. Eating a breakfast high in protein (which for VB6ers means whole grains, beans, peanut butter, tofu, and so on) will keep your hunger in check and rev up your engines so you can burn calories consistently for hours.

It's not that difficult, either, especially if you plan ahead and prepare a few items in advance. Make a big batch of something like cereal (page 138), pilaf (page 149), or grains (page 143) in advance and breakfast is as good as on the table when you wake up.

The key is to turn raw ingredients into meal components. With most recipes in this book—particularly the "Building Blocks" beginning on page 228—I've done some of the advance thinking and planning for you, pointing out dishes that work well when doubled or tripled and giving storage and reheating tips. All you need to do is pick a time during the week when you can dedicate a half hour to preparing breakfast items, and you're set for days—or longer.

SPICED APPLE JAM (WITH OR WITHOUT TOAST)

MAKES: 8 SERVINGS (ABOUT 2 CUPS)   TIME: ABOUT 1 HOUR AND 15 MINUTES

Most store-bought jams contain little or no fiber and loads of sugar—sometimes more sugar than fruit. Making jam at home allows you to control the amount of sugar (or skip it altogether) and play around with different combinations of fruits and nuts. This version has a spicy kick of ginger.

I don't peel the apples because I like skin (and the fiber), but if you prefer a smoother texture, go right ahead. When it's done, try spreading the jam on toast, spoon it over hot cereal (see page 143), or eat it straight like applesauce.

1½ pound apples, cored, peeled if you like, and roughly chopped

1 to 2 tablespoons sugar (optional)

2 tablespoons minced fresh ginger, or 2 teaspoons ground ginger

¼ teaspoon cinnamon

½ teaspoon salt

2 tablespoons fresh lemon juice

Whole-grain toast, for serving (optional)

1   Combine all the ingredients in a medium saucepan over medium heat. Bring to a boil, stirring occasionally.

2   Reduce the heat to a gentle bubble and cook, stirring occasionally and adding a bit more water if the mixture gets too dry, until it darkens and thickens, about 1½ hours.

3   Once the apples are quite soft you can mash them a bit with a fork or potato masher, if you like. Taste, and adjust the seasoning. Cool and refrigerate until you're ready to use. (It will keep for least a week.)

SPICED TOMATO JAM Substitute 1½ pounds chopped fresh or canned tomatoes (drained of their juice) for the apples, 1 teaspoon cumin for the cinnamon, and lime juice for the lemon juice. Add 1 minced jalapeño or a dash of cayenne if you want a little extra heat. Proceed with the recipe.

NUTRITIONAL INFO (¼ cup with 1 slice whole wheat toast):
Calories: 184 • Cholesterol: 0mg • Fat: 3g • Saturated Fat: 0g • Protein: 4g • Carbohydrates: 38g • Sodium: 283mg • Fiber: 5g • Trans Fat: 0g • Sugars: 13g

BROILED NUTTY APPLES

MAKES: 4 SERVINGS   TIME: 20 TO 30 MINUTES

Broiling is a fast and clever trick for turning common fruit into dessert, as well as an excellent way to prepare fruit that may be less than perfect. Just a few notes: The fat brings out the flavor of the seasonings and helps them stick to the apples; coconut oil is particularly rich if you have it handy. And although the fruit will become sweeter as you cook it, you can always add a sweetener to satisfy your cravings. Spices, nuts, and herbs are surprisingly delicious companions here—even ones you associate with savory foods—so be sure to explore the ideas that follow the recipe. Finally, broiled fruit goes great with any cold cereal; Corny Hoecakes (page 151); Breakfast Pilaf, Sweet or Savory (page 149); or of course is great by itself as a snack or after a meal.

> 4 apples
>
> 4 teaspoons vegetable oil
>
> 1 teaspoon cinnamon
>
> ¼ teaspoon nutmeg
>
> ⅛ teaspoon cloves
>
> ½ teaspoon salt
>
> 2 tablespoons maple syrup or agave nectar (optional)
>
> ½ cup chopped nuts (like walnuts or pecans)

1 Turn on the broiler; the heat should be medium-high and the rack no closer than 4 inches from the heat source.

2 Halve the apples through the equator and scoop out the seeds with a spoon or melon baller. Rub them all over with some oil and put them cut side down on a rimmed baking sheet. Broil until the skins are blistered and you can insert a fork into the flesh, 3 to 8 minutes, depending on your broiler.

3 Meanwhile, combine the spices and a sprinkle of salt in a small bowl. Turn the apples over, sprinkle with the spice mixture, and drizzle with the syrup, if you're using it. Broil, cut side up, until the apples are golden and fully tender, another 2 or 3 minutes; sprinkle with the nuts and pass under the broiler again until they just begin to toast, no more than 1 minute. Serve warm or at room temperature.

BROILED NUTTY PEACHES Hazelnuts are nice here. Instead of the cinnamon, nutmeg, and cloves, try ½ teaspoon cardamom or ground ginger.

BROILED VANILLA-SCENTED PEARS Try almonds with this variation. Cut the pears lengthwise, then remove the cores. Instead of using spices and salt, mix the oil with 1 teaspoon vanilla extract before coating and broiling the fruit.

BROILED MINTY GRAPEFRUIT Pistachios and grapefruit are a great combo. Omit the salt. You only need to broil the cut side, so drizzle the tops with the oil, and the syrup if you're using it. Keep an eye on the grapefruit as it cooks and remove it as soon as the top darkens in spots.

BROILED MELON WITH BALSAMIC Pine nuts are ideal here. Cut watermelon, cantaloupe, or honeydew into 1-inch-thick slices, and remove the seeds and rinds. Omit the spices, but salt, oil, and broil the fruit as described above. Serve drizzled with a few drops of balsamic vinegar and lots of black pepper.

NUTRITIONAL INFO *(apples with syrup and walnuts):*
Calories: 260 • Cholesterol: 0mg • Fat: 15g • Saturated Fat: 1g • Protein: 3g • Carbohydrates: 3g • Sodium: 246mg • Fiber: 6g • Trans Fat: 0g • Sugars: 24g

---

MORE WAYS TO FLAVOR BROILED NUTTY APPLES
Once you turn over the apples, sprinkle on any combination of spices or herbs, such as one of the following:

- ¼ teaspoon each allspice, cardamom, cumin, black pepper, and red chile flakes
- ½ teaspoon vanilla extract
- 1 tablespoon fresh lemon or lime juice
- 2 tablespoons chopped basil, Thai basil, or mint
- 1 tablespoon chopped rosemary or lavender

TROPICAL TOAST

MAKES: 4 SERVINGS   TIME: ABOUT 45 MINUTES

Bright orange juice and creamy coconut milk make a much more interesting custard for French toast than regular milk. A warm fruit topping made with fresh pineapple and shredded coconut adds sweetness and eliminates the need for loads of maple syrup and powdered sugar.

If you've got a juicer, try substituting fresh pressed pineapple juice for the orange juice here. And feel free to substitute any other fruit—berries, bananas, or stone fruit—for the pineapple.

½ cup freshly squeezed orange juice

½ cup coconut milk

1 teaspoon vanilla extract

¼ teaspoon salt

¼ teaspoon cinnamon or ⅛ teaspoon cloves

8 slices whole-grain bread

2 tablespoons shredded unsweetened coconut

2 cups chopped fresh pineapple

1 Heat the oven to 450°F. Whisk together the orange juice and ¼ cup of the coconut milk in a bowl, and stir in the vanilla, salt, and spice.

2 Put the bread on a rimmed baking sheet and brush both sides with the orange juice and coconut milk mixture until you've used it all. Bake until the tops are golden, 10 to 15 minutes, then turn the slices and bake until the second side is golden, 10 to 15 minutes more. (The bread should get a little crisp on top, but not crunchy all the way through.)

3 Meanwhile, put the coconut in a dry skillet over medium-high heat. Cook, stirring occasionally, until lightly toasted, 3 or 4 minutes, then transfer to a small bowl. Add the pineapple to the skillet and cook, stirring once in a while, until it's caramelized, 8 to 10 minutes. Return the coconut to the skillet and add ½ cup water and the remaining coconut milk, stirring to scrape any browned bits off the bottom of the skillet. Cook until the liquid reduces to a sauce as thick or thin as you like, 2 to 6 minutes. Spoon the sauce over the toast, and serve.

NUTRITIONAL INFO *(2 slices with topping)*:
Calories: 393 • Cholesterol: 0mg • Fat: 13g • Saturated Fat: 8g • Protein: 9g •
Carbohydrates: 64g • Sodium: 447mg • Fiber: 8g • Trans Fat: 0g • Sugars: 15g

BREAKFAST PILAF, SWEET OR SAVORY

MAKES: 4 SERVINGS   TIME: 45 TO 60 MINUTES

If you think you don't have the time to make hot cereal, think again. Yes, this takes a while, but most of the cooking here is unattended, and if you make double (or triple) batches, you can do the actual cooking once and reheat servings in the microwave all week long.

Rice is wonderful in the morning, but you can use quinoa or cracked wheat here without changing the technique at all. Steel-cut oats are good, too. Any of these will be ready with just 20 to 25 minutes of cooking time in Step 3.

I encourage you to try the savory variation and, for more grain and stir-in ideas, see the sidebar.

> 1 tablespoon olive or vegetable oil
>
> 1⅓ cups any long- or short-grain brown rice
>
> ½ teaspoon salt
>
> ¼ teaspoon each cinnamon, nutmeg, and ginger
>
> 2 tablespoons maple syrup
>
> 3 cups fruit, chopped if necessary
>
> ½ cup chopped fresh mint, for garnish (optional)

1 Put the oil in a large, deep skillet or medium saucepan over medium heat. When it's hot, add the rice. Cook, stirring, until the kernels are glossy, completely coated with oil, and have started to color, 3 to 5 minutes.

2 Add a pinch of salt and the spices and cook, stirring, until fragrant, about 1 minute. Add 1¾ cups water, the syrup, and half of the fruit: stir once or twice, and bring to a boil. Lower the heat so the mixture bubbles gently and cover the pan.

3 Cook until most of the liquid is absorbed and the rice is just tender, 20 to 40 minutes, depending on the rice. Uncover, stir in the remaining fruit and half of the mint, if you're using it. Replace the lid, and remove from the heat. Let the pilaf rest for at least 5—or up to 20—minutes. Taste and adjust the seasoning. Fluff the mixture with a fork and serve, topped with the remaining mint.

SAVORY BREAKFAST PILAF WITH SOY SAUCE AND CHERRY TOMATOES (Don't knock it 'til you try it!) Skip the spices and sugar. Substitute halved cherry tomatoes for the fruit, and chives or cilantro for the mint. Stir in 1 table-spoon soy sauce along with the liquid in Step 2 and add half of the cherry tomatoes. Continue with the recipe, stirring in the rest of the tomatoes and chives in Step 3. Pass more soy sauce at the table for drizzling.

HOT-AND-SWEET BREAKFAST PILAF Skip the sugar. Substitute 1 table-spoon dried chiles or 1 chopped fresh hot chile (like jalapeño or serrano) for the spices and add 1 chopped bell pepper and 1 chopped yellow onion along with the rice in Step 1.

NUTRITIONAL INFO *(with mixed fruit):*
Calories: 343 • Cholesterol: 0mg • Fat: 6g • Saturated Fat: 1g • Protein: 6g •
Carbohydrates: 68g • Sodium: 255mg • Fiber: 7g • Trans Fat: 0g • Sugars: 13g

MORE WAYS TO VARY BREAKFAST PILAF
Oatmeal is the go-to grain at breakfast, but it's only one of several options. As mentioned above, steel-cut oats, quinoa, and cracked wheat are all excellent substitutes. But don't stop there. Millet, farro, and kasha offer completely different flavors and chew, and take just a few minutes longer to cook. On days when you have more time, go for a big batch of longer-cooking grain, like wild rice, wheat berries, hulled barley, or hominy, which all have a satisfying hearty chew.

Even whole wheat couscous works well in this recipe, especially with dried fruit and spices like cinnamon and allspice. You need to make some adjustments, though: In Step 2, after you cover the pan, remove it from the heat and let it sit for 10 minutes, then continue with the recipe.

The stir-ins for this pilaf are only limited by what you've got handy (and what you think qualifies as breakfast—though this will probably change the longer you're eating VB6). Fresh and dried fruit, nuts, warm spices, and sweetener are typical breakfast flavorings, but if you're willing to go savory, a whole new world opens up. Try aromatics like onions, shallots, scallions, leeks, ginger, or lemongrass; any chopped fresh herbs or vegetables; or intense flavor boosters like olives, dried tomatoes, nuts, or even a spoonful of salsa or last night's leftover vegetables, slaw, or salad.

CORNY HOECAKES

MAKES: 4 SERVINGS   TIME: 30 MINUTES

A spin on New England johnnycakes, the quintessential pioneer food, these are like griddled cornbread but better. The simplicity of the batter makes it a perfect foil for any number of added ingredients and seasonings. The cornmeal version relies on corn kernels for crunch; the whole wheat variation uses fresh chopped fruit (you can also use fruit in place of corn in the main recipe). These reheat well, wrapped in foil and warmed at 300°F for 15 minutes.

Serve with Fruit Compote (page 230), Spiced Apple Jam (page 145), fresh chopped fruit, shredded coconut, chopped nuts, maple syrup, salsa, chopped herbs, or roasted, steamed or sautéed veggies. Or serve them as a bread-like accompaniment to soups and stews.

> 1½ cups cornmeal (fine or medium grind)
>
> 1 teaspoon salt
>
> 1½ cups boiling water, plus more as needed
>
> 3 tablespoons olive oil
>
> 1 cup fresh or frozen corn kernels

1   Heat the oven to 200°F. Combine the cornmeal and salt in a medium bowl. Gradually pour in the boiling water, whisking constantly. Let the mixture sit until the cornmeal absorbs the water, 5 to 10 minutes. Stir in half of the oil and a little more boiling water, a little at a time, until the batter is pourable. Fold in the corn kernels.

2   Put a large skillet or griddle, preferably cast iron or nonstick, over medium heat. When a few drops of water dance on the surface, add a thin film of the remaining oil. Working in batches, spoon in the batter, making any size cakes you like; they will be thinner than pancakes. Cook until bubbles appear and burst on the tops and the undersides are golden brown, 3 to 5 minutes; turn and cook on the other side until golden, another 2 or 3 minutes more. Transfer the cooked cakes to the warm oven and continue with the next batch, adding more oil to the skillet if necessary. Serve warm.

WHOLE WHEAT HOECAKES WITH FRUIT Substitute whole wheat flour for the cornmeal and 1 cup chopped firm fresh fruit (like berries, apples, pears, bananas, mango, or pineapple) for the corn kernels.

FLUFFY HOECAKES For a little rise in either the main recipe or the variation, add 1½ teaspoons baking powder to the bowl with the cornmeal or flour and salt.

NUTRITIONAL INFO *(served plain):*
Calories: 297 • Cholesterol: 0mg • Fat: 13g • Saturated Fat: 2g • Protein: 5g • Carbohydrates: 42g • Sodium: 509mg • Fiber: 4g • Trans Fat: 0g • Sugars: 3g

ADDITIONS
After you mix the batter, try stirring in one or more of these ingredients to load up your hoecakes:

- ½ cup chopped fresh herbs, like parsley, mint, basil, or cilantro; or 1 tablespoon fresh rosemary, thyme, oregano
- ½ cup chopped scallions
- 1 jalapeño, seeded and minced
- A few cloves of roasted garlic
- 1 cup chopped cooked greens, squeezed dry
- ¼ shredded unsweetened coconut
- 1 cup chopped fresh fruit
- ½ cup chopped nuts

TURKISH BREAKFAST

MAKES: 8 SERVINGS   TIME: 20 MINUTES WITH PRE-COOKED OR CANNED CHICKPEAS

Standard breakfast fare in the Middle East, this also makes a great snack or appetizer. The bean mixture is essentially hummus and variations on that theme. Garnish the plate with celery, fennel, carrots, or any other vegetables (or fruits; watermelon is quite common). Make a large batch and keep it for later. Or add more vegetables for dipping, and you've got perfect party food.

> 2 cups cooked or canned chickpeas, drained (reserve the liquid if you cooked them)
>
> 2 tablespoons olive oil
>
> 2 tablespoons tahini
>
> 3 tablespoons fresh lemon juice
>
> 1 teaspoon paprika or cumin (or both)
>
> 1½ teaspoons salt, plus more to taste
>
> Black pepper to taste
>
> 6 tomatoes, cored and sliced
>
> 1 cucumber, peeled if you like and sliced
>
> ½ cup green or black olives, pitted
>
> ¼ cup chopped fresh parsley
>
> Whole-grain toast, cut into triangles, for serving

1   Combine the chickpeas, 1 tablespoon of the oil, the tahini, lemon juice, paprika, and salt in a food processor or blender and puree until very smooth, adding some chickpea cooking liquid or water if necessary. Taste and adjust the seasoning.

2   Arrange the tomato and cucumber slices on a large plate or platter: add the olives and a large dollop of the bean mixture. Sprinkle everything with salt and pepper, drizzle with the remaining oil, and garnish with the parsley. Serve with the toast.

TUSCAN BREAKFAST Omit the tahini, spice, tomatoes, and cucumbers; increase the olive oil to 4 tablespoons. Instead of the chickpeas use white beans. In Step 1, add 1 tablespoon minced garlic and 1 teaspoon chopped fresh rosemary. Continue with the recipe and serve with the olives, segments from 6 oranges, 1 bulb sliced fennel, and the toast.

TEX-MEX BREAKFAST Omit the tahini, spice, cucumbers, and olives; increase the olive oil to 4 tablespoons. Instead of the chickpeas, use black beans and substitute lime juice for the lemon juice. In Step 1, add ½ teaspoon chili powder and ½ teaspoon cumin. Taste and adjust the seasoning, and serve with the tomatoes, 1 cup sliced radishes, chopped fresh cilantro, and warm or dry-toasted corn tortillas.

NUTRITIONAL INFO *(about ⅓ cup with 1 slice whole-wheat toast):*
Calories: 299 • Cholesterol: 0mg • Fat: 12g • Saturated Fat: 2g • Protein: 10g • Carbohydrates: 42g • Sodium: 768mg • Fiber: 8g • Trans Fat: 0g • Sugars: 7g

SCRAMBLED TOFU WITH SPINACH

MAKES: 4 SERVINGS   TIME: 20 MINUTES

In this hearty morning scramble, tofu takes the place of eggs. Since tofu is undeniably bland, it's important to ramp up the seasonings a bit. I like to use spinach, but any leafy greens will work. Other options: sliced mushrooms, leeks, cabbage, and asparagus; chopped broccoli, cauliflower, Brussels sprouts, and zucchini; or grated winter squash and root vegetables. This scramble makes an ideal lunch, too.

> 2 tablespoons vegetable oil
>
> 1 large onion, chopped
>
> 1 tablespoon chopped garlic, or more to taste
>
> 1 teaspoon salt, plus more to taste
>
> Black pepper to taste
>
> 1 tablespoon red chile flakes, or 1 or 2 fresh hot red chiles (like serrano or Thai), minced
>
> 1½ pounds fresh spinach, trimmed and rinsed well
>
> 1½ pounds firm or silken tofu, drained and patted dry

1   Put the oil in a large skillet over medium heat. When it's hot, add the onion and garlic and sprinkle with salt; cook until the onion is translucent and the garlic is soft, 3 to 5 minutes.

2   Add the chiles and cook, stirring, until fragrant, less than a minute. Raise the heat to medium-high and add the spinach and ¼ cup water. Sprinkle with salt and pepper and cook, stirring occasionally, until the spinach is wilted and fairly dry, 5 to 8 minutes.

3   Crumble the tofu into the pan and stir, using a spatula to scrape the bottom of the pan and combine the tofu and vegetables; adjust the heat as necessary to avoid burning. When the mixture starts to stick to the pan, it's ready: Taste and adjust the seasoning, and serve hot or warm.

SCRAMBLED TOFU WITH TOMATOES Use 2 pounds chopped tomatoes instead of the spinach. In Step 2, be sure to cook the tomatoes until they're dry before adding the tofu. Then continue with the recipe.

NUTRITIONAL INFO *(with firm tofu):*
Calories: 224 • Cholesterol: 0mg • Fat: 13g • Saturated Fat: 1g • Protein: 14g • Carbohydrates: 177g • Sodium: 727mg • Fiber: 5g • Trans Fat: 0g • Sugars: 5g

8

Lunch Recipes

Most of America's favorite midday meals are anything *but* vegan: burgers, of course, and deli sandwiches, meat-and-cheese–stuffed burritos, pizza—you know. For a "lite" meal, we might do chicken Caesar salad (which can weigh in at more than 1,000 calories). This makes lunching VB6 challenging, at least at first, especially because it's the meal we're most likely to eat away from home.

The alternative is not rabbit food but real food, and the recipes here offer a wide range of lunchtime options. With them and a few key strategies, you're set for every situation from office potluck or fancy lunch out with your boss to dining alone at your desk, or even a picnic with friends or family.

Your style of lunch can stay pretty much the same; all that changes is the food on your plate. If you eat sandwiches, go right ahead; start with the ideas on page 169. Eat out a lot? See the important tips on page 161. Into leftovers? (So am I.) On page, 157, I help take you beyond simply reheating (not that there's anything wrong with that) to show how you can "repurpose" dishes into entirely new meals.

VB6 lunches are tasty, varied, and satisfying alternatives to a pastrami sandwich. You'll enjoy a world of soups and salads, stir-fries and pastas, pitas and hummus, pizzas, and all sorts of international foods. As a reward for this discipline, you'll feel more energetic and less bogged down after lunch.

By the way, once in a long while, I *do* have that pastrami sandwich, and you may do the same. No big deal: You can balance it with a vegan dinner later. But if you're like me, you'll also find that these indulgences quickly become rare. When you base lunch on vegetables, you just feel too good in the afternoons.

LEFTOVERS FOR LUNCH

No matter where you work, lunch is the ideal opportunity to make a delicious meal out of food tucked away in the fridge. And once you start cooking and eating VB6, you'll always have plenty of beans, grains, and vegetables—raw and cooked—ready, wherever you need to go.

One key is to start thinking of food preparation in terms of components—there's a reason the last recipe chapter is called "Building Blocks"—and not just finished dishes. When you do, you'll top a bowl of greens with last night's cold roasted vegetables and cooked black beans from the weekend, and call it salad: While the coffee is brewing, you'll throw that stir-fry from a couple of days ago and the remaining brown rice into a container to nuke at the office. Spread a sandwich with pureed leftover veggies, toss beans, grains, and veggies into soups, warm up last night's tomato sauce with some grains, or bake it with some veggies— many things are possible, and good.

Another important tactic is to make large quantities of dishes that reheat especially well, like soups or stews. In this chapter—and throughout Part Two—I point out which recipes are best for this.

About storing and reheating: Invest in a wide-mouth thermos and some microwave-safe glass or silicone containers, or carry food in sealable bags and reheat meals in the microwave on plates. (Some plastic vessels are safer than others. Those that contain a chemical called bisphenol A—or BPA, for short—may become toxic, especially when heated.) Many lunch dishes can just be taken out of the fridge an hour or two before your break and enjoyed at room temperature.

GREEN SALAD WITH MACERATED FRUIT AND NUTS

MAKES: 4 SERVINGS   TIME: 30 MINUTES

I love fresh fruit in salads, especially the way the juices ooze flavor into the dressing. And this recipe changes with every season: Use berries and stone fruits in summer, apples and pears in fall, citrus and pineapple in winter, mangos and papaya in spring. Try dried fruit in the winter, too, but use no more than 1 cup—it's far more calorie dense than its fresh counterparts.

2 tablespoons any wine or balsamic vinegar

3 tablespoons olive oil

1 shallot or ½ red onion, minced

1 teaspoon salt, plus more to taste

Black pepper to taste

1½ pounds fresh or frozen fruit

10 cups mixed salad greens, torn into bite-size pieces

1½ cup nuts (like pecans, almonds, walnuts, or pistachios)

1   Put the vinegar, oil, shallot, salt, and some pepper in a large bowl and whisk until well combined.

2   Peel and core the fruit if necessary and remove any seeds or pits. If large, cut the fruit into ½-inch chunks. Add the fruit to the bowl along with any juice that may have accumulated. Toss to coat and let sit at room temperature for 5 to 10 minutes.

3   Add the greens and nuts, and toss until everything is evenly coated with dressing. Serve immediately.

NUTRITIONAL INFO *(made with peaches and pecans)*:
Calories: 448 • Cholesterol: 0mg • Fat: 39g • Saturated Fat: 4g • Protein: 7g • Carbohydrates: 26g • Sodium: 521mg • Fiber: 8g • Trans Fat: 0g • Sugars: 17g

LENTIL SALAD

MAKES: 4 SERVINGS   TIME: 30 MINUTES WITH COOKED OR CANNED BEANS

Try this once and you'll make it forever, probably never the same way twice. Lentils cook fast (see page 237), but feel free to substitute any kind of cooked, frozen, or canned bean here. If you toss them in the dressing while they're still warm, they'll absorb the flavor of the dressing beautifully.

Try any combination of chopped fresh vegetables, greens, or herbs; figure about 6 cups total.

> 1 tablespoon Dijon or other good-quality mustard, or to taste
>
> 2 tablespoons any wine or sherry vinegar
>
> 4 tablespoons olive oil
>
> 1 teaspoon salt, plus more to taste
>
> Black pepper to taste
>
> 4 cups cooked or canned lentils or any other beans, drained
>
> 3 large ripe tomatoes, chopped
>
> 1 large cucumber, peeled, seeded, and chopped
>
> 1 cup chopped carrots or radishes
>
> 1 cup chopped celery or fennel
>
> ½ cup chopped red onion
>
> ¼ cup chopped fresh parsley or dill

1 Put the mustard, vinegar, oil, and salt and a sprinkle of pepper in a large bowl. Add 2 tablespoons of water and whisk until well combined.

2 Add all of the remaining ingredients to the bowl and toss until coated with dressing. Taste and adjust the seasoning, and serve. (To make this salad ahead: Combine everything except the tomatoes and parsley; cover and refrigerate for up to a day, and let it come back to room temperature before serving.)

NUTRITIONAL INFO *(using carrots and celery):*
Calories: 425 • Cholesterol: 0mg • Fat: 16g • Saturated Fat: 2g • Protein: 21g • Carbohydrates: 53g • Sodium: 1052mg • Fiber: 20g • Trans Fat: 0g • Sugars: 11g

EASIEST VEGETABLE SOUP

MAKES: 4 SERVINGS   TIME: 45 TO 60 MINUTES

Make this with just about any vegetable you want—really. I like a combination of longer-cooking firm vegetables and quicker-cooking soft ones, but suit yourself. For that matter, you don't even need to use a combination of vegetables; if you like, just pick one or two (you're aiming for about 6 cups of vegetables overall), bearing in mind that beans, corn, or peas will add texture and body, making the soup more satisfying.

> 3 tablespoons olive oil
>
> 1 large onion, chopped
>
> 1 tablespoon minced garlic
>
> ¼ cup tomato paste
>
> 1 teaspoon salt, plus more to taste
>
> Black pepper to taste
>
> 6 cups vegetable stock or water
>
> 3 cups chopped firm vegetables (like carrots, winter squash, cauliflower, broccoli, or root vegetables)
>
> 3 cups chopped soft vegetables (like zucchini, bell peppers, green beans, or any greens)
>
> 3 cups cooked or canned beans, or fresh or frozen corn kernels or peas
>
> ½ cup chopped fresh basil, for garnish

1   Put the oil in a large pot or Dutch oven over medium-high heat. When it's hot, add the onion and garlic. Cook, stirring occasionally, until they begin to soften, 3 to 5 minutes. Stir in the tomato paste and cook until it dries out a bit, a minute or two. Sprinkle with salt and pepper.

2   Add the stock or water and scrape up any bits on the bottom of the pan. Add the firm vegetables. Bring to a boil, then adjust the heat so the mixture bubbles gently. Cook, stirring once in a while, until the vegetables are quite soft, 10 to 20 minutes, depending on the kinds you're using.

3   Add the zucchini or other soft vegetables, along with the beans, corn, or peas. Return to a boil, then lower the heat so the mixture bubbles gently. Cook, stirring once in a while, until everything is quite soft and

the soup begins to thicken, another 10 to 15 minutes. Stir in the basil, taste and adjust the seasoning, and serve.

EASIEST CREAMY VEGETABLE SOUP Carefully puree the finished soup in batches in a blender, or in the pot with an immersion blender, until it's a consistency you like, whether really smooth or quite chunky. Return to the pot and reheat, stirring occasionally.

NUTRITIONAL INFO *(with carrots, winter squash, zucchini, and white beans):*
Calories: 400 • Cholesterol: 0mg • Fat: 13g • Saturated Fat: 2g • Protein: 17g • Carbohydrates: 59g • Sodium: 1727mg • Fiber: 14g • Trans Fat: 0g • Sugars: 14g

---

EATING OUT FOR LUNCH

The average lunch menu contains way more meat and dairy than you would imagine, until you become conscious of it. On top of that, most restaurant portions are abnormally large—way bigger than what you'd prepare at home—and you'll be tempted to eat more as a result. But a casual lunch out doesn't need to be challenging; you can find good options almost everywhere. Some simple lunchtime tips:

1. Seek out salad bars where you can pile your plate high with vegetables; top with beans, nuts, seeds, or tofu. Drizzle with olive oil and vinegar or a little vinaigrette (*not* the creamy Caesar dressing or blue cheese) and you're set. Wait before getting seconds to give your body time to register what you ate. If you're actually still hungry, go back for more and again turn to vegetables first.

2. Make a meal of side dishes and vegetable soup or an appetizer or two.

3. Don't be afraid to make special requests. Usually you'll be asking to hold the cheese, mayo, butter, or meat. It's no big deal. And if it is, go elsewhere next time.

4. If you know you're eating somewhere that's not VB6 friendly, don't arrive hungry: Have a snack beforehand, then linger over a green salad.

5. Stick to water, coffee, or tea.

VEGETABLE MISO SOUP WITH TOFU AND RICE

MAKES: 4 SERVINGS   TIME: ABOUT 20 MINUTES

Traditional miso soup is ethereal, but you can transform this delicious and easy broth into a meal by tossing in rice and vegetables, and by ratcheting up the tofu. Buy refrigerated miso paste, which is better than shelf-stable varieties; the lighter the color, the milder the flavor. And be sure not to boil the soup after you've added the miso; extreme heat kills miso's beneficial enzymes and delicate flavor.

For the variations, canned or boxed vegetable stock is one way to go, but stock you make yourself will be so much better; see Fast and Flavorful Vegetable Stock on page 241.

> 2 pounds spinach, asparagus, snow peas, snap peas, or a combination, trimmed and cut into bite-size pieces as needed
>
> ½ teaspoon salt, plus more to taste
>
> ⅔ cup any miso paste, plus more to taste
>
> 1½ pounds firm tofu, cut into ½-inch cubes
>
> 3 cups cooked long- or short-grain brown rice (see page 235; optional)
>
> ¼ cup chopped scallions

1 Put 8 cups of water in a medium saucepan and bring to a boil over medium-high heat. Add the vegetables and salt and cook, stirring frequently until just barely tender, 3 to 7 minutes, depending on the vegetable. Turn off the heat.

2 Put about 1 cup of the cooking liquid in a small bowl and add the miso; whisk until smooth. Pour the miso mixture back into the saucepan and turn the heat to medium.

3 Add the tofu and the rice, if you're using it; stir once or twice and let sit for a minute, just long enough to heat everything through without letting the soup come to a boil. Taste and adjust the seasoning, adding more miso (whisked with some of the soup) and salt if necessary. Add the scallions and serve.

BROTHY SOUP WITH VEGETABLES AND TOFU Omit the miso and substitute vegetable stock (see the headnote) for the water. Serve with soy sauce and sesame oil for passing at the table.

EGG DROP SOUP WITH VEGETABLES For a quick, light dinner, omit the miso and tofu and substitute vegetable stock (see the headnote) for the water. While the vegetables are cooking in Step 1, beat 4 eggs well with a whisk. When the vegetables are tender, add the eggs to the soup in a steady stream, stirring constantly, and keep stirring until the eggs are cooked, just a couple of minutes. Serve with soy sauce and sesame oil for passing at the table.

NUTRITIONAL INFO *(with spinach, asparagus, and rice):*
Calories: 551 • Cholesterol: 0mg • Fat: 19g • Saturated Fat: 3g • Protein: 42g • Carbohydrates: 62g • Sodium: 2074mg • Fiber: 14g • Trans Fat: 0g • Sugars: 6g

GREENS AND BEANS SOUP

MAKES: 8 SERVINGS   TIME: 1½ TO 2 HOURS, LARGELY UNATTENDED

Greens and beans is among my favorite combinations, and you'll never run out of options. Start with dried beans if possible (use any you like; see page 236); their cooking liquid is deeply flavorful and gives the soup a rich texture. (To use canned or pre-cooked beans, follow the tofu variation below, using 8 cups of beans.)

I like hearty greens here, like kale or collards, cooked until tender, but not to the point of disintegrating; you could also use broccoli raab, escarole, spinach, or cabbage. Just make sure to either remove any thick stems (larger than ¼ inch) or chop them up and give them about 10 minutes in the broth before adding the leaves, so everything becomes tender at the same time. For a thicker, heartier broth, mash some of the beans with a potato masher before adding the greens; or puree half of them in a blender or food processor and add back to the soup.

Note that it's just as easy to make a big batch of this soup as a small one, so you can double the recipe and freeze serving-size containers to bring to the office.

> ¼ cup olive oil
>
> 1 large onion, chopped
>
> 2 tablespoons minced garlic
>
> ¼ teaspoon red chile flakes (optional)
>
> 2½ cups dried beans, any kind, rinsed, picked over, and
>   soaked if you have time
>
> 2 teaspoons salt, plus more to taste
>
> Black pepper to taste
>
> About 3 pounds kale, collard greens, broccoli raab, or
>   escarole (see the headnote), washed and roughly chopped

1 Put the oil in a stockpot over medium-high heat. When it's hot, add the onion and garlic. Cook, stirring occasionally, until they begin to soften, 3 to 5 minutes. Add the chile flakes if you're using them.

2 Add the beans, 3 quarts water, and the salt, and bring to a boil. Adjust the heat so the soup bubbles gently, and cover partially. Cook, stirring occasionally, until the beans are tender but still intact (anywhere from

30 to 90 minutes depending on the type of bean and whether or not you soaked them).

3   Return the soup to a boil, sprinkle with pepper, and stir in the greens. Partially cover and cook, stirring once or twice and adding more water if necessary to keep the mixture soupy, until the greens are tender, 10 to 20 minutes depending on the kind you use. Taste and adjust the seasoning, and serve.

GREENS AND TOFU SOUP Substitute 2 blocks firm tofu (about 2 pounds), cubed, for the beans. Instead of water, use vegetable stock (see page 241 for a recipe.) In Step 2, add the stock to the softened onions and garlic and bring to a boil; reduce the heat a bit, stir in the tofu and the greens, and cook, stirring occasionally, until the greens are tender, 10 to 20 minutes.

NUTRITIONAL INFO *(with white beans and kale):*
Calories: 384 • Cholesterol: 0mg • Fat: 9g • Saturated Fat: 1g • Protein: 20g • Carbohydrates: 62g • Sodium: 567mg • Fiber: 21g • Trans Fat: 0g • Sugars: 1g

STEWED TOMATOES AND BEANS

MAKES: 4 SERVINGS   TIME: 30 MINUTES

Try this the next time you have a craving for pasta and sauce; the beans cook in a classic tomato sauce until they become soft and slightly creamy. It's incredibly satisfying, and you can make it even more so by tossing it with whole wheat couscous or spooning it over brown rice.

2 tablespoons olive oil

1 onion, chopped

1 red or green bell pepper, chopped

1 tablespoon minced garlic

1 28-ounce can whole tomatoes, with their juice

4 cups cooked or canned beans, any kind, drained

1 teaspoon salt, plus more to taste

Black pepper

¼ cup chopped fresh cilantro or parsley, for garnish

1   Put the oil in a large skillet over medium-high heat. When it's hot, add the onion, bell pepper, and garlic. Cook, stirring occasionally, until they begin to soften, 3 to 5 minutes.

2   Add the tomatoes, beans, and the salt and some pepper. Adjust the heat so the mixture bubbles steadily. Cook, stirring occasionally, until the tomatoes break down, the beans begin to get soft and creamy, and the mixture begins to thicken, 10 to 15 minutes. If the mixture looks too thick, stir in a splash of water. (You can make the beans ahead to this point: Cover and refrigerate for up to 3 days, then gently reheat before proceeding.)

3   Taste and adjust the seasoning and serve, garnished with the herb.

TOMATOES AND GREEN BEANS Trim 1½ pounds green beans, but leave them whole. If you like the beans very tender, add them at the beginning of Step 2, as you would the cooked beans; for crisp-tender beans, wait to add them until the tomato sauce has cooked for 10 minutes. (This method also works with cauliflower, broccoli, or zucchini.)

NUTRITIONAL INFO *(with pinto beans):*
Calories: 371 • Cholesterol: 0mg • Fat: 9g • Saturated Fat: 1g • Protein: 18g • Carbohydrates: 58g • Sodium: 1179mg • Fiber: 19g • Trans Fat: 0g • Sugars: 8g

CHICKPEA RATATOUILLE

MAKES: 4 SERVINGS   TIME: ABOUT 1½ HOURS, LARGELY UNATTENDED

Classic ratatouille—a mixture of summery vegetables stewed with olive oil and herbs—is stellar and satisfying on its own. Add chickpeas (or cannellini, or lima beans) and you have a super-hearty main dish. Eggplant, zucchini, and peppers are the usual vegetables, but consider alternatives like roughly chopped hearty greens—escarole or kale, for example. Just be sure to keep the tomatoes for moisture.

> 1 pound eggplant (smaller ones are better), peeled if you like, and cut into large chunks
>
> ¾ pound zucchini, cut into large chunks
>
> 1 pound Roma (plum) tomatoes, cored and chopped, or 1 28-ounce can, drained
>
> 1 onion, sliced
>
> 2 red or yellow bell peppers, cored, seeded, and sliced
>
> 5 garlic cloves, halved
>
> 1 teaspoon salt, plus more to taste
>
> Black pepper to taste
>
> 4 tablespoons olive oil
>
> 3 cups cooked or canned chickpeas, drained
>
> 1 tablespoon chopped fresh thyme or rosemary, or ½ cup chopped fresh basil or parsley

1   Heat the oven to 425°F. Combine all the ingredients except the oil, chickpeas, and herbs in a large roasting pan. Drizzle with the oil and toss to combine.

2   Transfer to the oven and roast, stirring occasionally, until the vegetables are lightly browned and tender and some water has released from the tomatoes to create a sauce, 30 to 40 minutes.

3   Add the chickpeas, stir, and return to the oven until the beans heat through, 5 to 10 minutes. Add the herbs and stir. Taste and adjust the seasoning and serve hot, warm, or at room temperature.

NUTRITIONAL INFO:
Calories: 435 • Cholesterol: 0mg • Fat: 19g • Saturated Fat: 3g • Protein: 15g • Carbohydrates: 56g • Sodium: 803mg • Fiber: 18g • Trans Fat: 0g • Sugars: 17g

CREAMED MUSHROOMS ON TOAST

MAKES: 4 SERVINGS   TIME: 30 TO 45 MINUTES

Mashed white beans and a little water take the place of dairy here to thicken and enrich sautéed mushrooms. The flavor is more interesting than cream, the texture heartier, and the nutrition comparison isn't even close. Serve as a side dish, or make this a meal by ladling over whole-grain toast or flatbread. It's also good wrapped in whole wheat tortillas, over brown rice, tossed with whole wheat pasta, or used to sauce roasted wedges of eggplant, cabbage, or cauliflower.

> 2 tablespoons olive oil
>
> 1½ pounds fresh mushrooms, stemmed, if necessary, and sliced
>
> 1 teaspoon salt, plus more to taste
>
> Black pepper to taste
>
> 2 cups cooked or canned white beans, drained
>
> 1 tablespoon minced garlic
>
> 1 tablespoon chopped fresh thyme or rosemary, or 1 teaspoon dried
>
> Whole-grain toast, for serving
>
> ¼ cup chopped fresh parsley, for garnish

1   Put the oil in a large skillet over medium heat. When it's hot, add the mushrooms, sprinkle with the salt and some pepper, and cook, stirring occasionally, until the mushrooms have released their liquid, become tender, and the pan is beginning to dry out again, 10 to 15 minutes.

2   Meanwhile, puree the cooked beans in a food processor or blender with ½ cup water and let the machine run until the mixture is smooth. Stop to scrape down the sides and puree again. The mixture should thickly coat the back of a spoon. If not, add more water, 1 tablespoon at a time.

3   Add the garlic and thyme to the mushrooms along with ¼ cup water. Let the liquid bubble and evaporate for 1 minute, stirring the bottom of the pan to scrape up any browned bits, then add the bean mixture.

4   Cook, stirring occasionally, until the mixture becomes thick and saucy; add a few drops more water if it starts to stick to the pan. Taste and adjust the seasoning and serve on one or two slices of toast, garnished with the parsley.

CREAMED GREENS ON TOAST Substitute 1½ pounds leafy greens (such as spinach, escarole, or chard), roughly chopped, for the mushrooms. In Step 1, add ½ cup water to the pan along with the salt and pepper and continue with the recipe.

CREAMED BRUSSELS SPROUTS ON TOAST Trim 2 pounds Brussels sprouts instead of the mushrooms and cut them in half. Cook them as described in step 1, except add ½ cup water to the pan along with the salt and pepper. Continue with the recipe.

NUTRITIONAL INFO *(with 1 slice whole wheat toast):*
Calories: 367 • Cholesterol: 0mg • Fat: 11g • Saturated Fat: 2g • Protein: 17g • Carbohydrates: 56g • Sodium: 875mg • Fiber: 10g • Trans Fat: 0g • Sugars: 5g

ALTERNATIVE SANDWICHES

If your idea of lunch is a deli sandwich, you can still love VB6. You only need to adjust your mind-set a bit. Here are some tips to help take your thinking in a vegan direction:

Choose a vehicle: Some pre-sliced commercially prepared breads are more nutritious than others. Buy true whole-grain bread—the first ingredient on the label is your clue—or use whole wheat pita or whole wheat flour tortillas. To minimize the quantity of bread, consider open-face sandwiches on focaccia or whole-grain crackers like Wasa or RyVita; the recipe on page 243 is a great base for open-face sandwiches. Toasting the bread makes it sturdier for travel.

Choose a smear: Mashed beans or avocado, ground nuts, blended tofu, or pureed roasted vegetables will add substance and help keep things together. Season your spreads generously with fresh herbs or interesting spice blends, and add a little olive or sesame oil. You'll never miss the mayo.

Choose a filling: Now you're ready for raw or cooked vegetables and greens. Try to avoid anything that's too wet; this is why cooked— especially roasted or grilled—vegetables work especially well. (If you use boiled vegetables, which are also great, squeeze the water out of them first.) Finely chop or slice them into thin planks so they'll stay put. Thin slices of tofu (or the Tofu Jerky, page 189) can make a hearty meat alternative without resorting to heavily processed soy products. Add some lettuce or tomato (or not) and you're all set.

BLACK BEAN TACOS WITH TANGY CABBAGE

MAKES: 4 SERVINGS   TIME: 30 TO 45 MINUTES

The texture of lightly mashed, roasted beans mimics that of meat and is just as satisfying and hearty; filled with crunchy, cool, refreshing cabbage and a load of veggies, these are super tacos.

8 6-inch corn or whole wheat tortillas

3 tablespoons olive oil

2 cups cooked or canned black beans, drained

1 tablespoon minced garlic

1 tablespoon chili powder

½ teaspoon cumin

1 teaspoon salt, plus more to taste

Black pepper to taste

4 cups shredded green cabbage

1 red bell pepper, chopped

1 fresh hot green chile (like jalapeño or serrano), minced

¼ cup chopped scallions

Juice of 2 limes

½ cup chopped fresh cilantro

1   Heat the oven to 400°F. Coat a rimmed baking sheet with 1 tablespoon of the oil. Stack the tortillas and wrap them in aluminum foil. Combine the beans, garlic, chili powder, cumin, half of the salt, and some pepper in a bowl. Mash the mixture with a fork or potato masher; it should still be chunky.

2   Spread the mixture out on the prepared pan, drizzle with another tablespoon of oil, and roast, stirring a few times, until the beans are crumbly and crisp in places, 15 to 20 minutes. Transfer the tortillas to the oven with the beans for their last 5 minutes of cooking.

3   Meanwhile, put the cabbage, pepper, chile, scallions, lime juice, cilantro, remaining tablespoon oil and ½ teaspoon salt, and some pepper in a large bowl and toss to combine. Taste and adjust the seasoning. Divide the beans among the warm tortillas; top with the cabbage and serve.

NUTRITIONAL INFO *(2 tacos):*
Calories: 408 • Cholesterol: 0mg • Fat: 14g • Saturated Fat: 2g • Protein: 15g •
Carbohydrates: 62g • Sodium: 588mg • Fiber: 18g • Trans Fat: 0g • Sugars: 28g

---

SUBSTITUTIONS

Instead of the cabbage salad ingredients, try using any of the following
raw fruits and vegetables; figure 3 to 4 cups, alone or in combination:

Kale, shredded	Radishes, sliced	Butternut squash,
Red onions, thinly	Avocado, chopped	grated
sliced	Zucchini, grated and	Mangos, chopped
Fresh corn kernels	squeezed dry	Peaches, chopped
Tomatoes, chopped	Beets, grated	Jalapeños, sliced
Cucumbers,		thinly
chopped		

ONE-POT PASTA AND VEGETABLES

MAKES: 4 SERVINGS   TIME: 30 TO 45 MINUTES

Cooking pasta like risotto—the so-called absorption method—is effi-cient and delicious. Make sure you stir frequently, especially if you use long pasta, as it's more likely to get stuck together. (Breaking it into pieces, long considered heresy, also helps.) Once the pasta has begun to soften, but before it's fully tender, stir in any vegetables you like (see list below). I like to add parsley, too; other fresh herbs are also great.

> 4 tablespoons olive oil, plus more as needed
>
> 2 celery stalks, trimmed and chopped
>
> 1 carrot, chopped
>
> 1 onion, chopped
>
> 1 tablespoon minced garlic
>
> 1 teaspoon salt, plus more to taste
>
> Black pepper to taste
>
> ½ pound whole wheat cut pasta; or strands, broken into 2-inch pieces
>
> ½ cup dry white wine or water
>
> 4 to 5 cups vegetable stock (see page 241) or water
>
> 6 cups chopped raw vegetables (see the list below)
>
> ½ cup chopped fresh parsley

1   Put 2 tablespoons of the oil in a large, deep skillet over medium heat. When it's hot, add the celery, carrot, onion, and garlic, the salt, and some pepper. Cook, stirring occasionally, until the celery and carrots soften and the onion is translucent, 8 to 10 minutes.

2   Add the pasta and cook, stirring frequently, until it is glossy and starts to smell toasted, 2 to 3 minutes. Add the wine; stir and let the liquid bubble away.

3   Add the stock or water a ladleful at a time, stirring every minute or so until the liquid is almost evaporated and the pasta is just starting to stick. Add another ladleful of stock and continue to cook, stirring and adding stock as each addition is absorbed. Keep the heat medium to medium-high and stir frequently. Begin tasting the pasta 10 minutes after you add it; you want it to be just softening with a tiny bit of

crunch, which could take as long as 15 minutes, depending on the shape you've used.

4 Before the pasta is quite done, start stirring in the vegetables, beginning with the firmest (see the list below), and cook, adding more stock if the pan gets too dry, until they're nearly tender (by this time the pasta should be tender but not mushy). Stir in the parsley and the remaining 2 tablespoons oil. Taste and adjust the seasoning, and serve.

ONE-POT ASIAN NOODLES AND VEGETABLES Reduce the salt to ¼ teaspoon. Substitute soba or brown rice noodles (broken into pieces) for the whole wheat pasta, and peanut or vegetable oil for the olive oil. In Step 1, add 1 tablespoon minced ginger along with the garlic and use ¼ cup soy sauce mixed with ¼ cup water instead of the wine. Garnish with ¼ cup chopped scallions and toasted sesame seeds or chopped peanuts, if you like.

NUTRITIONAL INFO *(with broccoli):*
Calories: 444 • Cholesterol: 0mg • Fat: 16g • Saturated Fat: 2g • Protein: 13g • Carbohydrates: 62g • Sodium: 1126mg • Fiber: 5g • Trans Fat: 0g • Sugars: 7g

SUBSTITUTIONS
Stir in any combination of the following vegetables, sliced or chopped, in Step 4; this list is in order of firmest to most tender. Until you get the hang of it, here's a rough idea of when to add some examples: cauliflower or green beans at 12 minutes; zucchini or asparagus after 15; greens or bell peppers after 17. (You can also use pre-cooked or leftover vegetables, instead of raw: Wait until the pasta is almost entirely cooked, then stir them in at the last minute, and cook just long enough to warm through.)

Cauliflower	Broccoli	Fennel
Brussels sprouts	Zucchini	Spinach, kale or
Cabbage	Leeks	other greens
Eggplant	Asparagus	Fresh or roasted
Green beans	Tomatoes	bell peppers

SMASHED AND LOADED SWEET POTATOES

MAKES: 4 SERVINGS   TIME: ABOUT 1 HOUR, LARGELY UNATTENDED

Here's an updated version of the once-ubiquitous stuffed baked potato, made with nutritious, delicious, and colorful sweet potatoes. Veer the toppings toward the sweet or the savory, as you like. (See the list opposite for some ideas.)

You can cook the potatoes by either method well in advance, if you like. You can even refrigerate the cooked potatoes for a day or two. Then reheat them in a microwave for a couple of minutes before moving to Step 2.

4 large sweet potatoes, peeled

2 tablespoons olive oil

1 teaspoon salt, plus more to taste

Black pepper to taste

Any ingredient(s) from the list that follows, alone or in combination

1   Heat the oven to 425°F. Put the potatoes on a rimmed baking sheet, rub with some of the olive oil, and sprinkle all over with the salt. Roast the potatoes until a skewer or sharp knife inserted into one meets almost no resistance, 40 to 50 minutes. Or, put them on a plate, partially cover, and microwave on high for at least 10 minutes and up to 20 minutes, turning them over halfway through.

2   Once the potatoes are cool enough to handle, cut them in half and smash them a bit with a fork or potato masher; sprinkle with salt and pepper and drizzle with the remaining olive oil. Top with ingredients from the list below (or whatever you have handy) and serve.

NUTRITIONAL INFO *(with pine nuts, bell pepper, garlic, and balsamic):*
Calories: 410 • Cholesterol: 0mg • Fat: 27g • Saturated Fat: 3g • Protein: 6g • Carbohydrates: 40g • Sodium: 577mg • Fiber: 6g • Trans Fat: 0g • Sugars: 13g

SWEET AND SAVORY TOPPINGS FOR SMASHED AND LOADED SWEET POTATOES (FOR 4 POTATOES)

Up to 4 cups any cooked greens

1 cup roasted red bell peppers

2 cups black beans, cannellini, or chickpeas

2 cups peas or fava beans (frozen are fine)

2 cups corn kernels

½ to 1 cup chopped fresh herbs, like parsley, basil, or cilantro

Up to ¾ cup traditional pesto or herb puree

Up to ½ cup soy sauce

Up to ½ cup balsamic vinegar

Up to 2 tablespoons maple syrup

½ cup chopped olives

½ cup chopped nuts, like peanuts, pecans, or hazelnuts

Up to ¼ cup miso paste

2 tablespoons chopped chipotle in adobo

1 head roasted garlic

1 tablespoon ginger

1 tablespoon horseradish

2 teaspoons red chile flakes, paprika or cayenne

Hot sauce

EGGPLANT UN-PARMESAN

MAKES: 4 SERVINGS   TIME: ABOUT 1 HOUR

This take on eggplant Parmesan proves that (a) you don't need a lot of oil to cook eggplant, and (b) you don't need gobs of cheese to make it delicious. Try using zucchini or portobello mushrooms as variations, or serve the vegetables and tomato sauce over polenta for a more substantial meal.

If you can't find whole wheat breadcrumbs (panko-style are best), make your own by pulsing lightly toasted whole-grain bread in the food processor or blender.

> 2½ pounds eggplant
>
> 5 tablespoons olive oil
>
> 1¼ teaspoons salt, plus more to taste
>
> Black pepper to taste
>
> 1 onion, chopped
>
> 2 tablespoons minced garlic
>
> 2 28-ounce cans diced tomatoes, with their juice
>
> 1 cup chopped fresh basil leaves
>
> 1 cup whole wheat breadcrumbs, preferably coarse-ground

1 Heat the oven to 450°F and position two racks so that they've got at least 4 inches between them. Cut the eggplant crosswise into ½-inch-thick slices and arrange them on two rimmed baking sheets.

2 Use 2 tablespoons of the oil to brush the top of each eggplant slice and sprinkle them with ½ teaspoon salt and some pepper. Roast the eggplant until the slices brown on the bottom and sides, 10 to 15 minutes; turn and cook the other side until they're crisp in places and golden, another 5 to 10 minutes. When they finish cooking, remove them from the oven and lower the heat to 400°F.

3 Meanwhile, put 2 tablespoons of the oil in a large skillet over medium heat. When it's hot, add the onion, sprinkle with another ½ teaspoon of salt, and cook, stirring occasionally, until soft, 3 to 5 minutes. Add the garlic and cook, stirring, for 1 minute. Add the tomatoes and cook, stirring occasionally, until the tomatoes break down and the mixture comes together and thickens, 20 to 25 minutes. Taste and adjust the seasoning.

4   Cover the bottom of a 9 by 13-inch baking dish with about ½ inch of the tomato sauce. Nestle a layer of eggplant into the sauce and top with some of the basil. Cover with a thin layer of tomato sauce and repeat until all the eggplant is used up; reserve some of the basil for serving. Sprinkle with the breadcrumbs, the remaining ½ teaspoon salt, and lots of pepper, and drizzle with the remaining tablespoon of oil. Simmer the remaining sauce (you should have about 2 cups) over medium-low heat, stirring occasionally, while the eggplant bakes.

5   Bake until the breadcrumbs are golden and the sauce has thickened, 15 to 20 minutes; let rest for 10 minutes before serving. Serve hot, warm, or at room temperature, garnished with the remaining basil; pass the remaining sauce at the table (or refrigerate or freeze it for another use).

ZUCCHINI UN-PARMESAN Substitute 2 pounds zucchini (sliced lengthwise, preferably) for the eggplant and proceed with the recipe. Use mint instead of basil, if you like.

PORTABELLA UN-PARMESAN Use 1½ to 2 pounds portabella mushrooms instead of eggplant; remove their stems but leave them whole. Proceed with the recipe, only make one, not two layers. Use parsley instead of basil if you like.

EGGPLANT UN-PARMESAN WITH POLENTA Make a small batch of polenta (see page 235) and layer the tomato sauce, then the eggplant, the basil, and the polenta in a baking dish. Repeat until all the ingredients are used up. Top with breadcrumbs, if you like (it's not necessary). Bake as directed.

NUTRITIONAL INFO *(using all the sauce):*
Calories: 411 • Cholesterol: 0mg • Fat: 22g • Saturated Fat: 3g • Protein: 9g • Carbohydrates: 53g • Sodium: 1221mg • Fiber: 16g • Trans Fat: 0g • Sugars: 17g

NOW-OR-LATER VEGAN BURGERS

MAKES: 4 SERVINGS   TIME: 20 MINUTES WITH COOKED BEANS

These are the easiest and most versatile vegan burgers I know. Made with chickpeas the patties are golden brown and lovely; with black beans, much darker; with red beans, somewhere in between. Lentils give you a slightly meaty texture. In any case, they're great spiked with chili powder, cumin, or coriander. And note that you can replace the carrots with parsnips, sweet potatoes, rutabaga, turnips, winter squash—almost any root vegetable. For a knife-and-fork meal, try serving the burgers over salad greens or cooked vegetables.

Like almost all veggie burger mixtures, these will hold together a little better if you refrigerate them first. (Ideally you refrigerate both before and after shaping.) Once you've formed the patties, you can refrigerate them for a day or so or freeze them indefinitely.

2 cups cooked or canned black, white, or red beans, chickpeas, or lentils, drained, liquid reserved

1 small onion, roughly chopped

1 tablespoon chopped garlic

½ cup rolled oats

4 carrots, peeled and grated (about 1½ cups)

¼ cup chopped fresh parsley or cilantro

1 tablespoon chili powder or spice mix of your choice

1 teaspoon salt, plus more to taste

Black pepper to taste

¼ cup olive oil

8 slices whole wheat toast or toasted whole wheat hamburger buns

4 lettuce leaves

1 tomato (for 4 people)

½ red onion

4 tablespoons mustard

1   Combine the beans, onion, garlic, oats, carrots, parsley, chili powder, the salt, and some pepper in a food processor; pulse until combined but not pureed. Pinch a bit of the mixture to see if it holds together. If

not, add reserved bean liquid or water, 1 tablespoon at a time, until it does. If you have time, let the mixture rest for a few minutes before shaping the burgers.

2　Shape into four patties, about 1 inch thick. (Cover and refrigerate the burgers for up to several hours before continuing, or wrap and freeze; bring back to room temperature before cooking.)

3　Film the bottom of a large nonstick or cast-iron skillet with the oil and turn the heat to medium. When it's hot, add the burgers. Cook until browned on one side, 3 to 5 minutes; turn carefully and cook on the other side until firm, browned, and crisp in places, another 3 to 5 minutes. Serve hot or at room temperature, on the toast or buns, with the trimmings and mustard.

NUTRITIONAL INFO *(made with black beans and served as a sandwich with all the trimmings)*:
Calories: 530 • Cholesterol: 0mg • Fat: 22g • Saturated Fat: 3g • Protein: 14g • Carbohydrates: 74g • Sodium: 1043mg • Fiber: 12g • Trans Fat: 0g • Sugars: 9g

BAKED FALAFEL WITH TAHINI SAUCE

MAKES: 8 SERVINGS   TIME: 45 MINUTES, PLUS UP TO 24 HOURS TO SOAK CHICKPEAS

Falafel is easy: just soak raw chickpeas until they're soft enough to grind in the food processor, combine with some spices, shape, and bake. The baking makes lighter falafel, but they're just as crunchy as deep-fried.

This makes a big batch, which is fine, since you can refrigerate the leftovers for several days, or freeze them for a couple of months. To reheat, wrap them in foil and bake at 350°F until they're hot throughout, 15 to 30 minutes depending on whether they were frozen.

Here are some serving suggestions: Make a sandwich with half a whole wheat pita, lettuce, tomatoes, cucumbers, and other raw vegetables, then drizzle with sauce. Or add lemon juice to the sauce and eat on top of a green salad, using the tahini for dressing.

1¾ cups dried chickpeas

2 garlic cloves, chopped

1 small onion, quartered

1 tablespoon cumin

Scant teaspoon cayenne, or to taste

1 cup chopped fresh parsley or cilantro

1½ teaspoons salt, plus more to taste

½ teaspoon black pepper, plus more to taste

½ teaspoon baking soda

1 tablespoon fresh lemon juice

4 tablespoons olive oil

½ cup tahini

1   Put the chickpeas in a large bowl and cover with water by 3 or 4 inches—the beans will triple in volume as they soak. Soak for 12 to 24 hours, checking once or twice to see if you need to add more water to keep the beans submerged. (If the soaking time is inconvenient for you, just leave them in the water until they're ready; you should be able to break them apart between your fingers.)

2   Heat the oven to 375°F. Drain the chickpeas and transfer them to a food processor with the garlic, onion, cumin, cayenne, herb, 1 teaspoon of salt, pepper, baking soda, and lemon juice. Pulse until everything is minced but not pureed, stopping the machine

and scraping down the sides if necessary; add water tablespoon by tablespoon if necessary to allow the machine to do its work, but keep the mixture as dry as possible. Taste and adjust the seasoning, adding more salt, pepper, or cayenne as needed.

3   Grease a large rimmed baking sheet with 2 tablespoons of the oil. Roll the bean mixture into 20 balls, about 1½ inches each, then flatten them into thick patties. Put the falafel on the prepared pan and brush the tops with the remaining 2 tablespoons oil. Bake until golden all over, 10 to 15 minutes on each side.

4   Meanwhile, whisk the tahini and remaining salt with ½ cup water in a small bowl until smooth. Taste and adjust the seasoning and serve the falafel drizzled with the sauce.

NUTTY FALAFEL Replace ½ cup of the beans with an equal amount of walnuts, almonds, peanuts, or hazelnuts (don't soak the nuts). Omit the cumin and cayenne and use the cilantro instead of the parsley or try a tablespoon or so of thyme leaves. Proceed with the recipe.

NUTRITIONAL INFO *(with 1 whole wheat pita):*
Calories: 502 • Cholesterol: 0mg • Fat: 20g • Saturated Fat: 3g • Protein: 18g • Carbohydrates: 68g • Sodium: 813mg • Fiber: 14g • Trans Fat: 0g • Sugars: 6g

9

Snack Recipes

Staying satisfied between meals is a big part of why VB6 works; I nibble all day long and when you are VB6 you probably will, too. But the differences between VB6 snacking and SAD snacking are profound.

There are days when I have a handful of nuts more than once, and I usually eat several pieces of fruit every day, some in the morning and some in the afternoon. If I'm feeling like I want something more substantial, I may eat last night's leftover roasted veggies or a small salad at 11 in the morning or 4 in the afternoon.

Still, what works for me might not work for you; your taste is not mine. That's why I'm including recipes for snacks that eat like treats. You're still better off reaching first for fruit, vegetables, and nuts, but I've got some indulgences here for you, too: VB6-style chips, jerky, bonbons, and more. I love these things, and I'm betting you will, too.

I suggest you bring your own snacks with you *everywhere*, so you'll never have the excuse that you had nothing "good" to eat and had to hit the vending machines. It's not a big deal to slip a couple of apples or oranges into your backpack or purse, stash nuts in the car, or carry whatever it is you think you might need. Really, it's the only way you stand a chance.

It helps to drink water, too, and to drink a glass of water when you start to feel peckish to make sure you're not confusing hunger with thirst.

TIPS FOR KEEPING SNACKS HANDY

I've touched on good snacking habits elsewhere, but here's a full rundown:

Keep a few pieces of washed fruit in a bowl on the counter. If it's there, you'll eat it when you're home and take it with you on your way out the door. And be sure to have plenty of backup in the fridge, and some frozen fruit tucked away, too.

Prep long-lasting vegetables. You'll use them for spontaneous meals, too. Trim and peel carrots, cut up celery sticks and cucumbers, trim radishes, and pluck florets off cauliflower or broccoli. Keep carrots, radishes, and celery in a bowl of water in the fridge; everything else goes in airtight containers. (For dips, see page 191.) Pickled cucumbers or vegetables, sauerkraut, and cooked salsas are also good for snacking, and keep a long time.

Prepare salad greens as needed. Buy head and loose-leaf lettuces, spinach, or other greens and rinse them as soon as you can. (The prewashed kind are undeniably convenient; I still give them a rinse to freshen them.) It takes 15 minutes to sock away enough for several salads. Store the greens in a salad spinner or in sealable plastic bags with paper towels.

Keep roasted or raw nuts around, at home and at the office. If you're worried about moderating how much you eat, pack them in handful-sized single servings.

Use the microwave. In the time it takes to nuke a Hot Pocket you can have steamed broccoli or leftover beans drizzled with olive oil; or you can reheat last night's leftovers, cook half a sweet potato, or defrost a handful or two of frozen blueberries.

Make the recipes here: Tortilla Crisps and Tofu Jerky (pages 192 and 189) are my favorites.

CARROT CANDY

MAKES: 4 SERVINGS   TIME: ABOUT 3 HOURS, LARGELY UNATTENDED

Here, you concentrate the sweetness of carrots by slow-roasting them until they're essentially dehydrated. The resulting "candy" is slightly chewy and slightly crisp—the perfect healthy snack to eat alone, or as a vehicle for dips.

You can use this technique on virtually any vegetable, alone or in combination. Thinly sliced fennel bulbs, beets, parsnips, celery root, and turnips all work great, as will cauliflower or broccoli florets. All will take somewhere between 2½ and 3 hours, depending on the cut and how dry the vegetables were to begin with. If you want something crunchy and salty, try the variation.

If you have the pans and oven space, make at least a double batch, using an assortment of vegetables. Store in an airtight container in the fridge for up to a week.

> 8 medium carrots (about 1 pound)
>
> 1 tablespoon olive oil
>
> ½ teaspoon salt

1   Heat the oven to 225°F. Peel the carrots and cut them into ⅛-inch coins. Toss them with the olive oil and salt, then spread on a baking sheet in a single layer. Cook until slightly shriveled, dehydrated, and sweet but still soft and chewy. You might have to move them or the pan around to ensure they don't burn or get too crisp.

2   Start testing the carrots after about 2 hours, and remove them from the oven when they're as chewy or crisp as you like, another 30 to 60 minutes. Cool thoroughly before storing in an airtight container.

KALE CHIPS LACINATO Also known as black kale or *cavalo nero*, this vegetable is best for this recipe, but any kind of sturdy greens, like collards or red kale, will work, too. Cut the leaves into 2- to 3-inch pieces, then toss them with the oil and 1 teaspoon of salt. Continue with the recipe, but reduce the cooking time to 35 to 45 minutes.

NUTRITIONAL INFO *(about 2 carrots)*:
Calories: 58 • Cholesterol: 0mg • Fat: 4g • Saturated Fat: 1g • Protein: 1g • Carbohydrates: 6g • Sodium: 284mg • Fiber: 2g • Trans Fat: 0g • Sugars: 3g

VEGAN SNACK FOOD AND MEAT SUBSTITUTES

As being a vegan becomes more mainstream, so has vegan junk food. But these hyper-processed animal-free products are barely preferable to their meaty counterparts. If you want cheese, wait until after 6 o'clock and have some of the real thing rather than loading up on a dairy-free substitute; ditto a hamburger. Not being a full-time vegan is a key advantage of VB6, but an equally important component is avoiding foods that have long lists of unrecognizable ingredients.

So before you turn to vegan snack food and meat substitutes, try tofu; the recipes on pages 189 and 193 are a good place to start.

And then if you like tofu, you might also try tempeh and seitan, which have been mainstays in vegetable-based diets for centuries, with good reason: They're real, they're satisfying, and they can be prepared in many of the same ways you would tofu or meat. Since they're still a little out of the mainstream, I'm not including any specific recipes for them, but here's a little info on each to encourage you to give them a try on your own:

Tempeh This strange-looking cake usually made from fermented soybeans and originally from Indonesia is no beauty, but it has a complex, slightly sour flavor that many people find delicious. Buy it in natural food stores, Asian markets, and some supermarkets, either fresh (usually vacuum sealed for a longer shelf life; once opened, it keeps for only a few days) or frozen. It's super-nutritious with lots of protein and fiber. My preferred way to eat it: crumbled and crisped in a hot skillet filmed with sesame or peanut oil (or a combination), then added to stir-fried vegetables.

Seitan This wheat food—made from gluten, the protein of the grain— offers a wonderfully chewy, meaty texture. (It's the original mock meat, and as high in protein as a chicken breast.) You can find it in the refrigerated section of natural food stores, Asian markets, and some grocery stores; buy it plain, not marinated. I like to put a little crust on seitan before tossing it in sauces or stir-fries by pan-searing, roasting, broiling, or even grilling it first.

ROASTED VEGETABLE SPREAD

MAKES: 8 SERVINGS   TIME: 30 TO 90 MINUTES, LARGELY UNATTENDED

Run into a snack like this while you're rummaging in the fridge and you'll look no further; it's fantastic, and works for virtually any vegetable. Eat as is, on whole-grain crackers or toasted bread, or spread on sandwiches. You can also serve this alongside simply cooked meat or chicken for your after-6 meal.

Cooking time will vary from one vegetable to the next: High-moisture items, like tomatoes or zucchini, should be roasted until the pan is almost completely dry. Root vegetables and tubers, like sweet potatoes and carrots, will take a while to get tender. Greens will be ready to puree in 20 to 30 minutes.

The variations are endless; to get started, see the list that follows.

   8 cups raw vegetables, cut into chunks of roughly equal size

   1 head garlic, cloves peeled but left whole (optional)

   Herbs or spices of your choice (optional; see the list that
      follows)

   ¼ cup olive or vegetable oil

   2 teaspoons salt, plus more to taste

   Black pepper to taste

1 Heat the oven to 375°F. Toss the vegetables and garlic with the oil
   and salt in a large bowl. Spread the mixture out on two rimmed
   baking sheets. Transfer the pans to the oven and roast, tossing every
   20 minutes or so, until the vegetables are tender, dry, and browned in
   places, anywhere from 20 minutes to 1 hour.

2 Cool, then transfer vegetables to a food processor or blender or
   smash with a fork or potato masher until they are as smooth or as
   chunky as you like. Add water if necessary, a tablespoon at a time.
   Taste and adjust the seasoning and store, covered and refrigerated,
   for up to a week. Reheat, if you like, before serving.

VEGETABLE SPREAD, FROM LEFTOVERS If the vegetables were cooked until tender, regardless of the method, this will work. Drain if necessary, and put the vegetables in a blender or food processor; pulse until they're the texture you like, adding a little water if necessary. If they weren't cooked in oil, add 1 or 2 tablespoons olive or vegetable oil and pulse again. Reheat or serve cold or at room temperature.

NUTRITIONAL INFO *(made with broccoli, salt, and pepper, alone, without bread or crackers):*
Calories: 96 • Cholesterol: 0mg • Fat: 7g • Saturated Fat: 1g • Protein: 3g • Carbohydrates: 7g • Sodium: 515mg • Fiber: 2g • Trans Fat: 0g • Sugars: 2g

SOME VEGETABLE AND SEASONING COMBO IDEAS
Roast as described in the recipe, adding the spices or nuts during the last 5 minutes of cooking. Then puree and stir in the remaining herbs or seasonings:

Broccoli or broccoli raab with pine nuts and saffron

Cauliflower and carrots, and onion with cumin

Tomatoes and garlic with fresh or dried thyme

Mushrooms with scallions and soy sauce

Sweet potatoes with pimentón (smoked paprika)

Zucchini with garlic, lemon zest, and mint

Spinach with nutmeg, hazelnuts, and balsamic vinegar

Fennel with orange zest

Leeks with mustard

Beets and pistachios

SPIKED GUACAMOLE

MAKES: 4 SERVINGS   TIME: 15 MINUTES

Avocados are full of nutrients and good-for-you fat, but they're also calorie dense, so I like to extend guacamole to turn it into a thick, rich snack with great crunch. Here the avocado is combined with tomato, radishes, and lettuce, but you can use thawed frozen peas or corn, chopped asparagus, jícama, even mango or peaches. Eat with oven-baked corn tortillas, whole-grain crackers, crudités (page 191), or in lettuce cups or on celery sticks.

> 1 ripe avocado
>
> 1 teaspoon minced garlic
>
> Juice and zest of 1 lime
>
> 1 tomato, chopped
>
> 1 scallion, chopped
>
> 5 or 6 radishes, chopped
>
> 1 cup shredded romaine or iceberg lettuce
>
> 1 fresh hot chile (like jalapeño), stemmed, seeded, and minced
>
> ¼ cup chopped fresh cilantro
>
> 1 teaspoon salt, plus more to taste
>
> Black pepper to taste

Mash the avocado in a large bowl until it's as smooth or chunky as you like. Stir in the remaining ingredients; taste and adjust the seasoning. Eat immediately or cover and refrigerate for up to a day. (After an hour or so it will start to darken a bit, but will still be fine to eat.)

DOUBLE GREEN GUACAMOLE Puree the avocado with 4 cups chopped steamed asparagus in a food processor. Season with salt and pepper and serve as directed in the headnote.

NUTRITIONAL INFO *(for the guacamole alone)*:
Calories: 104.36 • Cholesterol: 0mg • Fat: 7.6g • Saturated Fat: 1g • Protein: 2g • Carbohydrates: 9.9g • Sodium: 497mg • Fiber: 5.6g • Trans Fat: 0g • Sugars: 2.4g

TOFU JERKY

MAKES: 4 SERVINGS   TIME: ABOUT 1 HOUR, LARGELY UNATTENDED

Beef jerky is everywhere. Tofu jerky—oh, not so much. (You've probably never even heard of such a crazy thing.) It's great stuff, characteristically crusty and chewy. Most commercially made jerky, whether it starts with beef or soy-based meat substitutes, is loaded with additives and preservatives; here, you control all the ingredients.

> 1 pound firm tofu
>
> 1 tablespoon tomato paste
>
> 1 teaspoon soy sauce
>
> ¼ teaspoon liquid smoke
>
> 2 teaspoons brown sugar
>
> ½ teaspoon smoked paprika (pimentón)
>
> ¼ teaspoon ground Chinese five-spice

1 Heat the oven to 225°F. Line a baking sheet with parchment paper or a silicon mat. Cut the block of tofu in half through the equator and blot the halves dry. Then cut each half the long way into slices a bit thicker than ⅛ inch (you should have about 28 slices total), and lay them on the parchment (it's preferable if they're touching).

2 Bake the tofu for 30 minutes. Meanwhile, stir together the remaining ingredients with 1 tablespoon water. After 30 minutes, lightly brush the top side of the tofu with half of the sauce, and bake for another 15 minutes. Flip the slices and cook for another 30 minutes, then lightly brush the second side with more sauce and bake for another 15 minutes. The tofu should be chewy (not crunchy) and still very pliable.

3 Let the jerky cool completely (the slices will get a bit more crisp as they cool). Eat right away, or refrigerate in a sealed container for up to a week.

NUTRITIONAL INFO *(for a 7-slice serving):*
Calories: 94 • Cholesterol: 0mg • Fat: 5g • Saturated Fat: 1g • Protein: 10g • Carbohydrates: 5g • Sodium: 114mg • Fiber: 1g • Trans Fat: 0g • Sugars: 4g

EDAMAME

MAKES: 4 SERVINGS   TIME: 5 MINUTES

Edamame—young, green soybeans, still in their pods—are traditional in Japan, and are increasingly popular here. Lucky us, since they are nutritious, easy to find (especially frozen) and prepare, and super delicious. Though they're often served with just a sprinkling of salt, there are plenty of ways to jazz them up: toasted sesame seeds, sesame oil, soy sauce, rice vinegar, grated citrus zest, ground spices.

Any time you see fresh shell beans in the pod at your farmers' market—any kind—grab 'em. The cooking times may vary a little, but you can treat them exactly this way.

> 1 teaspoon salt, plus more to taste
>
> 1 pound fresh or frozen edamame in their pods
>
> Black pepper to taste

1 To boil the beans, bring a large pot of water to a boil and salt it. Add the edamame, return to a boil, and cook until bright green, 3 to 5 minutes; drain. To microwave the beans, put the edamame in a microwave-safe dish with ¼ cup water and a pinch of salt, partially cover, and microwave on high until bright green, 1 to 5 minutes, depending on your microwave power.

2 Sprinkle the edamame with the teaspoon salt, and a little or a lot of black pepper. Toss and serve hot, warm, or chilled (with an extra bowl on the side for the empty pods). To eat, split the shells open and pluck out the beans, or pop one end in your mouth and squeeze out the beans with your teeth.

EDAMAME OUT OF THE SHELL You can either shell them yourself or buy them already shelled. Cook according to Step 1. Put the shelled beans in a serving bowl and toss, if you like, with about 1 teaspoon of sesame oil. Sprinkle with the salt and pepper, and serve with toothpicks.

NUTRITIONAL INFO *(using salt in the boiling water and as seasoning):*
Calories: 125 • Cholesterol: 0mg • Fat: 5g • Saturated Fat: 0g • Protein: 12g • Carbohydrates: 10g • Sodium: 976mg • Fiber: 5g • Trans Fat: 0g • Sugars: 3g

CRUDITÉS WITH SOY DIPPING SAUCE

MAKES: 8 SERVINGS   TIME: 5 MINUTES, WITH PREPARED VEGETABLES;
UP TO 1 HOUR OTHERWISE

If you keep a variety of both cooked and raw vegetables handy, along with a jar of homemade dipping sauce, you don't have to wait for a party to enjoy this classic appetizer; instead, it becomes an everyday snack.

Cut the vegetables into pieces that are big enough to dip but small enough to eat in a bite or two. Cucumber, cherry tomatoes, radishes, celery, summer squash, jícama, fennel, and carrots are all good raw, as are thinly sliced beets, turnips, and other root vegetables. String beans, broccoli, cauliflower, Brussels sprouts, asparagus, and the like should be steamed or boiled, then shocked in a bowl of ice water to keep them crisp-tender.

Store fully prepped raw vegetables in cold water. Keep cooked vegetables in airtight containers.

¼ cup soy sauce

¼ cup chopped scallions

2 tablespoons lemon or lime juice

2 tablespoons toasted sesame seeds

2 tablespoons dark sesame oil

1 tablespoon minced ginger

3 pounds assorted raw and/or cooked vegetables

1 Whisk together the soy sauce, scallions, lemon juice, sesame seeds, sesame oil, and ginger in a small bowl with ¼ cup water.

2 Cut the vegetables any way you like and serve them with the sauce on the side for dipping.

CRUDITÉS WITH LEMON TOFU DIPPING SAUCE Whisk together 2 to 3 table-spoons fresh lemon juice, ⅓ cup silken tofu, 1 teaspoon minced garlic, and ¼ cup chopped fresh herbs, like parsley, basil, cilantro, or dill.

NUTRITIONAL INFO (with carrots, broccoli, zucchini, radishes, cherry tomatoes, and new potatoes):
Calories: 120 • Cholesterol: 0mg • Fat: 6g • Saturated Fat: 1g • Protein: 4g • Carbohydrates: 15g • Sodium: 449mg • Fiber: 4g • Trans Fat: 0g • Sugars: 4g

TORTILLA CRISPS

MAKES: 4 SERVINGS   TIME: ABOUT 30 MINUTES

Deep-fried tortillas aren't exactly diet food, and commercially made flavored chips are loaded with both chemicals and calories. But try this: Take fresh corn tortillas, smear them with a quickly seasoned tomato paste, and bake until crisp. As the tortillas crisp, the tomato topping intensifies; you're left with warm chips and "salsa" rolled into one.

> ¼ cup tomato paste
>
> 2 tablespoons olive oil
>
> 1 teaspoon chili powder
>
> ½ teaspoon salt, plus more to taste
>
> Black pepper to taste
>
> 8 small corn tortillas

1   Heat the oven to 350°F. Combine the tomato paste, olive oil, chili powder, salt, and some black pepper in a small bowl. Put the tortillas on a baking sheet (or two) and use your fingers or a brush to smear a thin layer of the tomato mixture onto the top of each.

2   Bake until the tortillas are as chewy or crisp as you like them and the tomato paste has darkened slightly, 20 to 25 minutes. Break the tortillas into pieces if you like. Serve warm or store in an airtight container at room temperature for up to a few days.

NUTRITIONAL INFO *(for 2 tortillas):*
Calories: 188 • Cholesterol: 0mg • Fat: 9g • Saturated Fat: 1g • Protein: 4g • Carbohydrates: 25g • Sodium: 413mg • Fiber: 4g • Trans Fat: 0g • Sugars: 2g

VEGAN "CREAMSICLES"

MAKES: 4 6-OUNCE FROZEN POPS   TIME: 5 MINUTES, PLUS ABOUT 4 HOURS
TO FREEZE

An amazing spin on the popular orange and vanilla Creamsicles, but these are super easy and free of corn syrup and additives. The secret ingredient is silken tofu, which is available in most supermarkets, fresh or in sealed boxes. It's the ideal replacement for yogurt, so I use it in smoothies (page 139) and anytime I want to add a tangy creaminess.

⅔ cup soft silken tofu

1⅓ cups fresh orange juice

2 tablespoons sugar

1 teaspoon vanilla extract

1   Put all the ingredients in a blender and puree until the mixture is smooth and the sugar is dissolved, 1 or 2 minutes.

2   Pour the mixture into plastic molds for making frozen pops, or if you don't have them, use paper cups; transfer them to the freezer. If you use cups, wait about 1 hour, then insert a wooden frozen-pop stick into each cup; it should stand upright. Continue freezing until the snacks are completely solid, another 2 or more hours. To release, run the mold under cool water for a few seconds to loosen them (or peel off the paper cup).

NUTRITIONAL INFO:
Calories: 93 • Cholesterol: 0mg • Fat: 1g • Saturated Fat: 0g • Protein: 3g •
Carbohydrates: 17g • Sodium: 3mg • Fiber: 0g • Trans Fat: 0g • Sugars: 15g

CHOCOLATY PINEAPPLE KEBABS

MAKES: 6 SERVINGS (12 SKEWERS)   TIME: ABOUT 3 HOURS, LARGELY UNATTENDED

Pineapple and chocolate combine to make an amazing treat. Drying out the pineapple concentrates its sweetness and makes it more chewy than juicy, while the cocoa powder on the outside adds a slightly bitter edge. The end result is a wonderful snack that can also double as dessert. Mangos and apples are other good fruits to try here; figure about 2 pounds of either.

> 12 wooden or metal skewers
>
> 1 large pineapple
>
> 2 tablespoons cocoa powder

1   Heat the oven to 250°F. If you're using wooden skewers, soak them in water for 20 to 30 minutes. Trim the top and bottom from the pineapple and cut it into quarters. Remove the tough core from each piece and separate the flesh from the skin with a serrated knife; cut out any remaining eyes. Cut the pineapple into 1½-inch chunks. (You should have about 6 cups.)

2   Thread the pineapple chunks onto the skewers; put the skewers onto a rack set over a sheet of parchment paper (or anything to catch the extra cocoa powder.) Pour the cocoa powder into a fine-mesh strainer and gently tap the side of the strainer to evenly dust the fruit all over, turning the skewers as necessary.

3   Put the rack on a baking sheet and transfer to the oven. Cook until the pineapple has shriveled and dried and the cocoa has darkened, 2½ to 3 hours. Let the skewers cool, then eat the pineapple immediately or remove from the skewers and store in an airtight container in the fridge for a day or two.

NUTRITIONAL INFO *(2 skewers):*
Calories: 87 • Cholesterol: 0mg • Fat: 1g • Saturated Fat: 0g • Protein: 2g • Carbohydrates: 23g • Sodium: 3g • Fiber: 4g • Trans Fat: 0g • Sugars: 15g

FROZEN BANANA BONBONS

MAKES: 8 SERVINGS   TIME: 30 MINUTES, PLUS TIME TO CHILL

This is a version of something you've probably loved for years: fruit dipped in chocolate. The best chocolate—for recipes as well as indulging—is dark chocolate with 60 percent or higher cocoa content. Bananas are my favorite here, but any fresh fruit or nuts will work equally well.

The trick lies in heating and cooling the chocolate to a specific temperature before you start dipping the bananas, a process called tempering. You'll need a candy or instant-read thermometer along with a double boiler or a bowl set over a saucepan of simmering water.

   8 ounces good-quality dark chocolate, finely chopped

   4 bananas, peeled and each cut into 8 chunks

1 Line a baking sheet with parchment paper. Melt 6 ounces of the chocolate in a small, clean metal or glass bowl set over simmering water, or in the top of a double boiler. When the chocolate reaches between 110 and 115°F on a candy thermometer, remove it from the heat.

2 Add the remaining chocolate to the bowl, stirring constantly with a rubber spatula until the chocolate reaches 82 to 84°F. Put the bowl back over the simmering water and bring the temperature back up to between 88 and 91°F. Remove it from the heat and start dipping the bananas: Use a fork to first coat each banana chunk about halfway, then give it a twirl and turn it upside down so the banana is almost entirely covered in chocolate. Put each bonbon on the prepared baking sheet to set the coating.

3 Repeat with the remaining chocolate and banana chunks, keeping the thermometer close so you can keep checking the temperature. If it drops below 88°F (which it probably will once or twice), put the bowl back over the simmering water until it returns to the 88 to 91°F range, then continue dipping.

4 Let the bananas cool until the chocolate has hardened, then freeze them on the pan. When they're hard, transfer them to an airtight container and store in the freezer for up to a couple of months.

NUTRITIONAL INFO (4 bonbons):
Calories: 217 • Cholesterol: 2mg • Fat: 11g • Saturated Fat: 6g • Protein: 2g • Carbohydrates: 28g • Sodium: 3mg • Fiber: 4g • Trans Fat: 0g • Sugars: 18g

10
Dinner Recipes

Reward time. After exercising that discipline all day, dinner is not only a time to unwind, enjoy the company of friends and family, and just relax; it's also a time to eat the food that you may have been craving all day long. Worrying about calories runs contrary to the spirit of the evening, and at 6:00 P.M. we can let the indulging begin.

You may find, though, as I did, that your definition of indulgence changes. When I first started VB6, I ate old style: fancy meals out, big dinners, burgers or pizza, desserts. But though I still eat all of those things, I do so a lot less frequently. After only a few weeks of VB6, my dinnertime cravings began to change: I just didn't need as much food to feel satisfied as I once had, and desserts were less of a turn-on; if I had them at all, I was happy with just a bite or two.

Ironically, it was dinnertime that most demonstrated that I'd shifted toward a more plant-based diet. And it happened painlessly, without my ever consciously thinking about it. Really.

And the recipes here reflect that: You probably have all the recipes you need for old-fashioned meals. The recipes here are more balanced, more in the flexitarian (or what I also call less-meatarian) mode: They're for omnivores, but omnivores who are increasing the amount of plants in their diets.

So what follows is a collection of versatile recipes that give you an idea of typical VB6 dinners. The food is familiar, satisfying, easy to prepare, and delicious. All include meat, poultry, fish, dairy, and fish, but their proportions to vegetables are turned upside down; the vegetables are the focus. But because it all feels like normal dinner fare, not much different from what you're accustomed to eating, you'll find these meals easy to love. And easy to cook.

Once you start eating from this chapter, you'll be pleasantly surprised by how much flavor just a few ounces of meat or a tablespoon of butter will add; just a bit contributes mightily to texture and flavor. When you're thinking of animal products as a garnish and as flavoring— as has been traditional in so many cultures of the world throughout time—just a few slices of bacon, two eggs, or a small hunk of grated Parmesan are a satisfying addition to your daytime fare of vegetables, beans, and grains. The stir-fry on page 198 and the frittata on page 201 are perfect illustrations of how "eating upside down" works.

STEAK AND BROCCOLI STIR-FRY

MAKES: 4 SERVINGS   TIME: 30 MINUTES

Once you learn one stir-fry, you pretty much have mastered the art, and you can make a different one every day of your life and never encounter a repetition unless you wanted to. (See sidebar, page 200.) This one works with just about any combination of vegetables and protein, which might be boneless chicken breasts or thighs, sturdy white fish, shrimp or squid, or pork shoulder. You could also skip the meat altogether and substitute tofu.

The other ingredients are equally flexible. I like broccoli here, but try, alone or in combination, bell peppers, cabbage, bok choy, fennel, spinach, snow peas or snap peas, asparagus, summer or winter squash, green beans, mushrooms, carrots, or cauliflower. For a change from rice, serve with whole-grain soba or rice noodles.

4 tablespoons vegetable oil

12 ounces beef flank or sirloin steak, very thinly sliced (easiest if you freeze the meat for 30 minutes)

1 teaspoon salt, plus more to taste

Black pepper to taste

2 tablespoons minced garlic

1 tablespoon minced ginger

1 tablespoon minced fresh hot chile (like jalapeño or Thai; optional)

1½ pounds broccoli, trimmed and cut into bite-size pieces

½ cup chopped scallions

2 tablespoons soy sauce, plus more to taste

Juice of 1 lime or ½ lemon (optional)

¼ cup chopped peanuts or cashews

3 cups cooked long- or short-grain brown rice

1 Put a large, deep skillet over high heat. When it's hot, add 1 tablespoon of the oil, swirl it around, and add the beef. Sprinkle with ½ teaspoon of the salt and some pepper, and cook, stirring occasionally, until the beef starts to brown, 3 to 5 minutes. Transfer the meat to a plate.

2   Add the remaining 3 tablespoons oil, then the garlic, ginger, and chile, if you're using it. After 15 seconds, add the broccoli and all but a handful of the scallions. Cook, stirring infrequently, until the broccoli is bright green and beginning to brown, 3 to 5 minutes. Add the remaining ½ teaspoon salt and ½ cup of water. Cook, stirring occasionally, until almost all the liquid has evaporated and the broccoli is almost tender, another minute or two more.

3   Return the meat to the pan along with the soy sauce and lime juice, if you're using it, and a little more water if the mixture is dry. Raise the heat to high and cook, stirring occasionally, until the liquid is reduced slightly. Stir in the peanuts, then taste and adjust the seasoning if necessary; garnish with the remaining scallions, and serve over the rice.

NUTRITIONAL INFO *(with ¾ cup brown rice):*
Calories: 572 • Cholesterol: 55mg • Fat: 28g • Saturated Fat: 5g • Protein: 31g • Carbohydrates: 54g • Sodium: 1510mg • Fiber: 10g • Trans Fat: 0g • Sugars: 6g

THE MASTER STIR-FRY FORMULA

This stir-fry is really a universal recipe: Once you get it, you can plug in any ingredients that you have handy. And every stir-fry need not be Asian; you can veer toward the Mediterranean (chicken, escarole, tomatoes, and garlic), Indian (lamb, okra, and curry powder), or even Mexican (beef, corn, poblano chiles, and lime), for example. Here are the steps:

1. **Cook some protein.** Get a skillet good and hot, add some oil, and then add thinly sliced or chopped meat, pork, poultry, tofu, bigger pieces of fish, whole scallops, mussels, shrimp, or clams (even in their shells). The times will vary but cook, stirring only to keep things from burning, until the food loses its raw color and is almost fully cooked; you'll add it back to the skillet at the end, so just shy of done is best. Empty the skillet and put it back on high heat.

2. **Cook the aromatics and vegetables.** Add a bit more oil to the skillet, immediately followed by fragrant ingredients like minced garlic, ginger, chiles, chopped onions, scallions, shallots, or leeks. This is when you have the opportunity to vary flavors. For example, if you're going for a Mediterranean approach, consider chopped olives, dried tomatoes, capers, or anchovies. Aromatics can burn quickly in a hot skillet so cook them only for about 15 seconds; then add the primary vegetables (see the recipe headnote for lots of ideas). Let the vegetables brown a bit before stirring and adding water, which helps them steam and makes a little sauce as they cook. Until you get the hang of improvising, keep checking their tenderness, adding water if necessary to keep the mixture moist. You want the vegetables just a little firmer than the way you want to eat them before continuing. Again, timing will vary, so use your judgment.

3. **Add the finishing touches.** Return the meat or other protein to the pan and add any liquid flavorings that you like: soy sauce, fish sauce, citrus juice, a splash of wine, beer, stock, or vinegar; you may need a little water as well. (Soy sauce will burn if the mixture gets too dry.) Let the liquid reduce a bit to thicken. Adjust the seasoning as you like, stir in any final additions, like nuts, sesame seeds, or herbs, and serve.

ZUCCHINI FRITTATA

MAKES: 4 SERVINGS   TIME: 30 MINUTES

I adore frittata, which is a rare, any-time-of-day dish—you can eat it when you make it, or at room temperature, or even cold, straight from the refrigerator.

Normally a frittata uses 2 eggs to each cup of vegetables, but VB6 style reverses that, using 1 egg to bind 2 cups of vegetables. Here I use zucchini, but you have lots of other options: spinach, chard, or broccoli raab; fresh or dried tomatoes; potato or sweet potato; asparagus; mushrooms; winter squash, carrots, or parsnips; even eggplant. The smaller you cut the vegetables, the sooner they'll be ready for the eggs; just make sure the pan juices have evaporated before adding them.

You can also make this frittata with 4 cups of cooked vegetables. Simply add them to the softened onion in Step 1; add the herbs if you like, and cook for just 2 or 3 minutes before adding the egg.

6 bacon slices, chopped

2 tablespoons olive oil

½ onion or 1 large shallot, sliced

4 zucchini, chopped (about 8 cups)

1 teaspoon salt, plus more to taste

Black pepper to taste

¼ cup fresh basil, mint, or parsley, or 1 teaspoon chopped fresh rosemary, thyme, or tarragon (optional)

6 large eggs

½ cup grated Parmesan cheese

1   Put the bacon in a large skillet over medium heat. Cook, stirring occasionally, until it has started to brown and become crisp, 5 to 10 minutes. Transfer the bacon to paper towels. Pour all but 2 tablespoons of the fat out of the skillet, and return the skillet to the heat.

2   Add the olive oil to the skillet. When the oil is hot, add the onion, and cook, stirring occasionally, until it softens, 3 to 5 minutes. Add the zucchini, sprinkle with ½ teaspoon salt and some pepper, raise the heat to medium-high, and cook, stirring occasionally, until it just

softens, 5 to 10 minutes. Adjust the heat so the zucchini dries and browns a little without scorching. When the zucchini is completely dry, turn the heat to low and add the bacon and the herbs, if you're using them. Stir until combined.

3   Meanwhile, beat the eggs with the remaining ½ teaspoon salt and some pepper, along with the cheese. Pour over the vegetables, tilting the pan to distribute them evenly. Cook, undisturbed, until the eggs are barely set, 15 to 30 minutes, depending on the size of your skillet. (You can set them further by putting the pan in a 350°F oven for a few minutes, or running it under the broiler for a minute or two.) Cut into wedges and serve hot, warm, or at room temperature.

NUTRITIONAL INFO:
Calories: 414 • Cholesterol: 314mg • Fat: 32g • Saturated Fat: 10g • Protein: 23g • Carbohydrates: 9g • Sodium: 1164mg • Fiber: 2g • Trans Fat: 0g • Sugars: 6g

CHOOSING CHEESE AND DAIRY
Once you start eating VB6-style, your dairy consumption will likely plummet, so you may as well enjoy it to the fullest and use the best full-fat cheeses, yogurt, and milk you can find. (It will be much more satisfying than that low-fat, high-processed stuff.) Look for products from animals that haven't been treated with a common hormone given to cows called rBST and haven't been injected with antibiotics, and instead choose products derived from animals that are raised in decent and humane conditions. Even if that means spending a little more per item for better quality, your overall dairy budget will be way lower.

BAKED ZITI WITH VEGETABLES AND CHEESE

MAKES: 4 SERVINGS   TIME: ABOUT 1 HOUR

Think of this as vegetable-heavy mac 'n' cheese or a deconstructed lasagna. In any case, it gives the satisfaction of a pasta and cheese dish, but with much more VB6-friendly proportions. You get more vegetables, just a little cheese, and fewer carbohydrates. The result is wonderful, and the vegetables perfectly complement that great toothsome texture of pasta. The recipe calls for fennel, but check out the list that follows for a variety of vegetables that can work the same way.

Since you can prepare this in advance, it's great for entertaining: Double the recipe and bake it in a 9 by 13-inch pan.

> 2 teaspoons salt, plus more to taste
>
> 4 tablespoons olive oil
>
> 1 small red onion, sliced
>
> 2 large fennel bulbs (about 1½ pounds), halved and thinly sliced
>
> 1 tablespoon minced garlic
>
> 1 teaspoon red chile flakes
>
> 1 28-ounce can tomatoes, chopped, with their juice
>
> Black pepper to taste
>
> 8 ounces whole wheat ziti or other large-cut pasta
>
> 4 ounces grated mozzarella cheese
>
> 4 ounces ricotta
>
> 1 cup grated Parmesan cheese

1   Bring a large pot of water to a boil and add 1 teaspoon salt. Heat the oven to 400°F and grease a 9 by 9-inch baking dish with 1 tablespoon of the olive oil.

2   Put the remaining 3 tablespoons oil in a large skillet over medium heat. When it's hot, add the onion, sprinkle with ½ teaspoon salt, and cook, stirring occasionally, until the onion is translucent, 3 to 5 minutes. Add the fennel, garlic, and red chile flakes, and cook until the fennel softens a bit, another 3 to 5 minutes. Add the tomatoes and remaining ½ teaspoon salt and the pepper and bring to a boil. Reduce the heat to a gentle bubble and cook, stirring occasionally, until the sauce thickens slightly, about 5 minutes.

3   Meanwhile, cook the pasta halfway through; start checking after 3 minutes; it should just be getting tender but still be quite chalky inside. Drain it, reserving about a cup of the cooking water. Toss the pasta with the sauce, mozzarella, and ricotta; add enough cooking water to make the mixture quite moist, but not soupy.

4   Spoon the mixture into the prepared pan. (You can make the recipe to this point up to a day in advance; cover and refrigerate, then bring it back to room temperature before proceeding.) Sprinkle with the Parmesan and bake until the top is browned and the sauce has thickened, 20 to 30 minutes. Let sit for 5 minutes before serving.

BAKED ZITI WITH VEGETABLES AND MEAT Substitute ½ pound ground beef or sausage for the ricotta and use mozzarella instead of the Parmesan if you like. Before adding the vegetables to the skillet in Step 2, add the meat to the hot oil and cook, stirring occasionally, until browned all over, 5 to 10 minutes; drain all but 3 tablespoons of the fat if necessary. Add the onion and fennel and proceed with the recipe.

BAKED ZITI WITH LEFTOVER VEGETABLES This is especially great if you have grilled or roasted zucchini, mushrooms, or eggplant in the fridge: Skip the fennel and figure 3 cups chopped or sliced cooked vegetables. In Step 2 cook the onion in the oil, then add the garlic and cook and stir for a minute or two before adding the tomatoes. After the sauce cooks and thickens a little, stir in the cooked vegetables and proceed with the recipe.

NUTRITIONAL INFO:
Calories: 565 • Cholesterol: 38mg • Fat: 27g • Saturated Fat: 9g • Protein: 23g • Carbohydrates: 64g • Sodium: 1,595mg • Fiber: 11g • Trans Fat: 0g • Sugars: 6g

SUBSTITUTIONS
Chop or slice about 1½ pounds of any of these vegetables into bite-size pieces, then add them instead of the fennel in Step 2.

Broccoli	Cabbage	Carrots
Broccoli raab	Escarole	Eggplant
Cauliflower	Chard	Bell peppers
Brussels sprouts	Spinach	Mushrooms

LOADED FRIED RICE

MAKES: 4 SERVINGS   TIME: 30 MINUTES

Restaurant fried rice usually consists of a huge pile of heavily oiled rice with scrambled eggs and a few token green peas. This version is different, a mixture that's heavy on vegetables, light on the rice (which is brown, not white), and full of flavor. Since fried rice is the ideal vehicle for whatever vegetables, meat, chicken, tofu, or seafood you have in the fridge, don't be afraid to make it up as you go.

A few tips: The best consistency comes from cold leftover rice. (If you cook a fresh batch and try to fry it without cooling it for a day, it will come out sticky and mushy.) And if you have other cooked whole grains in the fridge, use 'em instead.

And there's no need to confine yourself to the vegetables listed here. Chopped celery, tender greens, or frozen peas all cook in a flash; and if you want to use sturdier vegetables like asparagus, green beans, broccoli, or cauliflower, just cut them into very small pieces first. For the protein you can try flank or skirt steak, boneless and skinless chicken thighs, or firm or baked tofu (all cut into cubes or thinly sliced); sea scallops, sliced in half crosswise; or squid, cut into bite-size pieces.

> 3 tablespoons vegetable oil
>
> ½ cup chopped scallions or red onion
>
> 1 cup bean sprouts or thinly sliced cabbage
>
> 1 cup snow or snap peas
>
> 1 red bell pepper, chopped
>
> 1 celery stalk, chopped
>
> 1 carrot, chopped
>
> ½ teaspoon salt, plus more to taste
>
> Black pepper to taste
>
> 12 ounces peeled and chopped shrimp, or chopped pork loin (or a combination)
>
> 1 tablespoon minced garlic
>
> 1 tablespoon minced ginger
>
> 1½ cups cooked long-grain brown rice, preferably leftover and chilled

2 large eggs

¼ cup dry white wine or water

2 tablespoons soy sauce

1 tablespoon sesame oil

1   Put 1 tablespoon of the oil in a large skillet over high heat. When it's hot, add the scallions, bean sprouts, snow peas, bell pepper, celery, and carrot. Sprinkle with the ¼ teaspoon of the salt and some black pepper and cook, stirring occasionally, until the vegetables soften and begin to brown, 5 to 10 minutes. (Lower the heat a bit if they start to burn.) Remove the vegetables from the pan with a slotted spoon.

2   Add another tablespoon of oil to the pan, followed by the shrimp and/or pork; sprinkle with the remaining ¼ teaspoon salt. Cook and stir until the meat and chicken are no longer pink, 2 or 3 minutes. Add them to the vegetables. Put the remaining tablespoon of oil in the skillet, followed by the garlic and ginger. About 15 seconds later, begin to add the rice, a bit at a time, breaking up any clumps with your fingers and stirring it into the oil.

3   When all the rice is added, make a well in its center and break the eggs into it; scramble them a bit then mix them in with the rice. Return the meat and/or shrimp and vegetables to the pan and stir to combine. Add the wine and cook, stirring, until it evaporates, less than a minute. Add the soy sauce and sesame oil; taste, adjust the seasoning if necessary, and serve.

NUTRITIONAL INFO *(with pork and shrimp):*
Calories: 426 • Cholesterol: 173mg • Fat: 24g • Saturated Fat: 4g • Protein: 22g • Carbohydrates: 27g • Sodium: 987mg • Fiber: 4g • Trans Fat: 0g • Sugars: 5g

STEEL-CUT OATS, RISOTTO-STYLE

MAKES: 4 SERVINGS   TIME: ABOUT 1 HOUR

Classic risotto is made with rice, of course, but steel-cut oats (and other grains, too) also develop a luxurious creaminess while retaining terrific chew when cooked with this technique. As with classic risotto, you can flavor this with almost anything you like. See the lists on the following page for some of my favorite combinations or develop your own.

Note that if you leave out the Parmesan, this becomes a perfect VB6 lunch dish.

½ cup dried porcini mushrooms

1½ cups very hot water

4 to 5 cups vegetable stock (see page 241) or water

3 tablespoons olive oil

1 onion, chopped

About 1½ teaspoons salt, plus more to taste

1½ cups steel-cut oats

Black pepper to taste

½ cup dry white wine or water

2 cups sliced fresh shiitake or portabella mushroom caps

1 cup grated Parmesan cheese

¼ cup or more chopped fresh parsley

1 Soak the porcini mushrooms in the hot water until they soften a bit, at least 10 minutes. Put the stock in a medium pot over medium-low heat. Put 2 tablespoons of the oil in a large, deep skillet over medium heat. When it's hot, add the onion, sprinkle with ½ teaspoon of the salt, and cook, stirring occasionally, until it softens, 3 to 5 minutes.

2 Add the oats to the skillet and cook, stirring occasionally, until they're glossy and coated with oil, 2 to 3 minutes. Add the remaining teaspoon of salt and some pepper, then the white wine. Stir frequently and let the liquid bubble away. Lift the porcini out of the soaking liquid with a slotted spoon and chop them. Add the porcini to the grains and stir them in together with about 1 cup of their soaking liquid, pouring carefully to leave any sediment in the bowl.

3 Use a ladle to add ½ cup of the hot stock to the oats, stirring almost constantly. When the stock has just about evaporated in the skillet,

add more, and continue cooking and adding stock, ½ cup or so at a time, stirring after each addition. The mixture should be neither soupy nor dry. Stir frequently, keeping the heat at medium to medium-high; make sure the oats don't stick to the skillet. Begin tasting the oats 20 minutes after you have added them; you want them to be tender but still noticeably chewy; it will probably take around 30 minutes total cooking time to reach this stage.

4   Meanwhile, put the remaining tablespoon of the oil in a small skillet over medium-high heat. When it's hot, add the fresh mushrooms and cook, stirring occasionally, until lightly browned and almost crisp, about 10 minutes; remove from the heat and sprinkle with some salt. When the oats are ready, stir in the cooked mushrooms, half the Parmesan, and the parsley. Taste, adjust the seasoning, and serve immediately, passing the remaining Parmesan at the table.

NUTRITIONAL INFO:
Calories: 556 • Cholesterol: 22mg • Fat: 23g • Saturated Fat: 7g • Protein: 24g • Carbohydrates: 63g • Sodium: 1677mg • Fiber: 11g • Trans Fat: 0g • Sugars: 7g

SUBSTITUTIONS
Other grains to try, from quickest cooking to the slowest (the longer it takes to cook, the more stock or water you'll need to add):

Bulgur	Farro	Wheat berries
Quinoa	Kamut	Rye berries
Pearled barley	Brown rice	
Kasha		

Cook these vegetables on the side in Step 4; figure up to 4 cups total:

Asparagus	Green beans	Chopped greens
Snow peas	Lima beans	Cherry tomatoes
Artichoke hearts	Corn	Fennel
Fava beans	Peas	

To add meat or seafood, figure about 12 ounces. In Step 4, remove the fresh mushrooms from the pan and use the remaining fat in the pan to cook any of the following:

Ground beef	Boneless chicken	Squid
Sausage	Shrimp	Scallops

SHRIMP TABBOULEH

MAKES: 4 SERVINGS   TIME: 30 MINUTES

The traditional way to make this salad is with lots of herbs and tomatoes and only a small amount of bulgur; I like to include even *more* fresh vegetables. If you then add shrimp (or squid or chicken or whatever), you have a simply super main-course salad.

Substitute quinoa, steel-cut oats, or millet for the bulgur if you like; each brings its own characteristic flavor and texture. And be sure to dress the tabbouleh with lemon and olive oil while the grain is still warm, so it absorbs all the flavors and fluffs up a bit.

¾ cup medium-grind bulgur

¼ cup olive oil

Juice of 2 lemons, or to taste

1 teaspoon salt, plus more to taste

Black pepper to taste

1 pound cooked shrimp, chopped if large

3 tomatoes, chopped

1 cucumber, peeled, seeded, and chopped

1 bunch radishes, chopped

2 celery stalks, chopped

4 scallions, chopped

8 green olives, pitted and chopped

1 cup roughly chopped fresh parsley

1 cup roughly chopped fresh mint

1 Bring 1½ cups of water to a boil in a small pot. Remove from the heat, stir in the bulgur, and cover. Let sit until tender, 15 to 20 minutes. If any water remains in the bottom of the pot, strain the bulgur, pressing down on it with a spoon, or squeeze it dry in a cloth.

2 Toss the warm bulgur with the oil and lemon juice; add the salt and sprinkle with some pepper. (You can make the bulgur up to a day in advance. Cover and refrigerate; bring to room temperature before proceeding.)

3 Just before you're ready to eat, add the remaining ingredients and toss with a fork; taste, adjust the seasoning, adding more olive oil, lemon juice, or salt and pepper as needed, and serve.

NUTRITIONAL INFO:
Calories: 420 • Cholesterol: 239mg • Fat: 19g • Saturated Fat: 3g • Protein: 32g • Carbohydrates: 33g • Sodium: 1671mg • Fiber: 9g • Trans Fat: 0g • Sugars: 5g

SUBSTITUTIONS/ADDITIONS
Stir in any of the following ingredients instead of (or in addition to) the shrimp in Step 2. For vegetables, beans, and other protein, add up to 2 cups; for more calorie-dense foods like cheese, nuts, and seeds, use no more than 1 cup.

Chopped raw peppers	Shaved raw artichoke hearts	Crumbled feta or queso fresco
Thinly sliced fennel	Cooked white or fava beans or chickpeas	Mozzarella cubes
Thawed frozen corn kernels or peas		Chopped olives
Shredded raw cabbage	Chopped cooked meat, chicken, or seafood	Chopped almonds or other nuts
Chopped salad greens or spinach	Crumbled tofu	Sunflower, pumpkin, or sesame seeds
Roasted peppers		

FISHERMAN'S STEW

MAKES: 4 SERVINGS   TIME: ABOUT 1 HOUR

This hearty, classic Mediterranean vegetable and seafood stew—a kind of ratatouille meets bouillabaisse—comes together quickly. Saffron is optional (but very good), as is a slice of toasted crusty bread in the bottom of each bowl.

3 tablespoons olive oil

1 large fennel bulb, or 4 celery stalks, trimmed and thinly sliced; fronds or leaves reserved and chopped

2 red bell peppers, cored and thinly sliced

1 large red onion, thinly sliced

1 tablespoon minced garlic

1 teaspoon salt, plus more to taste

1 large pinch saffron (optional)

½ teaspoon red chile flakes or cayenne, or to taste

1 sprig fresh tarragon or thyme

Black pepper to taste

2 cups chopped tomatoes (canned are fine; drain them first)

12 ounces Yukon Gold or other all-purpose potatoes, peeled if you like, and cut into 1½-inch chunks

2 cups vegetable stock (see page 241) or water, plus more as needed

1 pound fish or shellfish (like thick white fish fillets, scallops, squid, or shrimp), peeled, skinned, boned, and cut into chunks as needed

2 carrots or parsnips, cut into thin coins

2 small zucchini, thickly sliced

4 thick slices whole-grain bread, toasted

1   Put the olive oil in a large pot over medium-high heat. When it's hot, add the fennel bulb, peppers, onion, garlic, salt, and saffron, if you're using it, and cook, stirring occasionally, until the vegetables have softened, 5 to 10 minutes. Add the red chile flakes, tarragon, and sprinkle with pepper. Cook and stir until fragrant, just another minute. Add the tomatoes and potatoes, and stock. Bring to a boil, reduce the heat so the liquid bubbles gently, and cover.

2   After about 20 minutes, lift the lid and stick a fork into a potato; if it's not yet beginning to get tender, cover and cook another 5 minutes. When the fork meets with just a little resistance, add the carrots and zucchini and adjust the heat so that the liquid again bubbles gently.

3   When the carrots and zucchini are nearly tender (after 6 to 8 minutes), add the seafood and cook until it's opaque and just cooked through, 2 or 3 minutes for shrimp, scallops, and squid, 4 to 6 minutes for thick fish fillets. Stir in the fennel fronds or celery leaves, then taste and adjust seasoning, adding lots of black pepper. Serve with or over the bread.

NUTRITIONAL INFO:
Calories: 482 • Cholesterol: 28mg • Fat: 16g • Saturated Fat: 2g • Protein: 26g • Carbohydrates: 61g • Sodium: 1186mg • Fiber: 11g • Trans Fat: 0g • Sugars: 14g

STEAMED VEGETABLES AND SEAFOOD IN PACKAGES

MAKES: 4 SERVINGS   TIME: 30 MINUTES

Cooking vegetables and fish in packages may sound a bit fussy, but really it's an efficient way to cook, with two huge bonuses: The packages are easy to assemble ahead of time for entertaining, and they make cleanup a snap. They're impressive-looking, too. Round out the meal with a big salad and some bread or cooked grain for soaking up the juices and you're in business.

You can use many different vegetables here, but since the fish cooks quickly, they should be tender to start out with and sliced thinly. I almost always add tomatoes, since the juices that they release during cooking create a wonderful sauce. Mushrooms, eggplant, and fennel are also great. The fish fillets or steaks should be 1 inch thick; salmon, halibut, or cod are all good choices. Or you can use shrimp, scallops, or even mussels and clams. (Figure about 3 pounds total for these mollusks; just double the size of the packages to accommodate them.) Chicken (cutlets or boneless thigh) work well, too.

> 2 zucchini, thinly sliced
>
> 2 red bell peppers, cut into strips
>
> 2 leeks (white part and some green), trimmed, well rinsed, and thinly sliced (sliced scallions or onions are also okay)
>
> 2 large ripe tomatoes, cored and thinly sliced
>
> 1 teaspoon salt
>
> Black pepper to taste
>
> 4 sprigs fresh thyme
>
> 4 1-inch-thick fish fillets or steaks (like cod, sea bass, halibut, or catfish), about 1 pound
>
> 4 tablespoons olive oil
>
> ¼ cup dry white wine or water

1   Heat the oven to 400°F. Cut foil into 4 rectangles of at least 18 by 12 inches, fold in half crosswise to crease, then open again like a book.

2   On one half of each rectangle, layer a portion of the zucchini, peppers, and leeks, and tomatoes, keeping the vegetables close to the center. Sprinkle with half the salt and some pepper and top with a sprig of thyme. Add a piece of fish and sprinkle with the remaining ½ teaspoon salt. Drizzle each serving with 1 tablespoon of the olive oil and 1 tablespoon of the wine. Seal the packages by enclosing the filling and rolling the edges together tightly. Transfer the packages to two rimmed baking sheets.

3   Bake the packages until the vegetables are tender and the fish is just cooked through (it's done when you can insert a thin-bladed knife through the foil into the fish without resistance), 15 to 20 minutes. Let the packages sit for a couple of minutes before cutting the tops open; be careful to avoid the steam when you do so. Serve immediately in the packages, or transfer to plates, with the juices poured over all.

NUTRITIONAL INFO *(with cod):*
Calories: 317 • Cholesterol: 49mg • Fat: 17g • Saturated Fat: 2g • Protein: 23g • Carbohydrates: 17g • Sodium: 570mg • Fiber: 4g • Trans Fat: 0g • Sugars: 9g

HURRY CURRY

MAKES: 4 SERVINGS   TIME: 40 MINUTES

A little bit of richness goes a long way in this spicy stew, a quick amalgam of stir-frying and braising. You can use any vegetable you like here; just remember that firmer vegetables take a little longer to get tender.

The directions provide guidance for a few options, and you can explore even more. But if you just want to throw everything into a pot and forget about it (also a great option), see the slow-cooker variation.

    2 tablespoons vegetable oil

    12 ounces boneless, skinless chicken thighs, cut into chunks
      or slices and blotted dry

    1 teaspoon salt, plus more to taste

    Black pepper to taste

    1 tablespoon minced ginger

    1 bunch scallions, white and green parts separated and
      chopped

    1 or 2 small dried hot red chiles (like Thai), or a pinch red
      chile flakes

    1 tablespoon curry powder

    1 cup vegetable stock (see page 241) or water, plus more
      as needed

    6 cups firm vegetables (like cauliflower, broccoli, Brussels
      sprouts, cabbage, carrots, zucchini, or eggplant), roughly
      chopped

    1 cup fresh or frozen peas, halved cherry tomatoes, or
      sliced okra

    ½ cup coconut milk

    ½ cup yogurt

    ½ cup chopped fresh cilantro, for garnish

    3 cups cooked short- or long-grain brown rice

1 Put a large, deep skillet over high heat. When it's hot add 1 tablespoon
   of the oil, swirl it around, and immediately add the chicken. Stir once,
   add the salt and sprinkle with pepper, and sear for a minute before
   stirring again. Cook, stirring occasionally, until the chicken has lost
   its pink color, 3 to 5 minutes. Remove from the pan and pour off all but
   1 tablespoon of the fat.

2 Add the remaining tablespoon of oil, the ginger, white parts of the scallions, chiles if you're using them, and curry powder, and cook, stirring, until fragrant, just a minute or so. Add the stock and the firm vegetables. Bring to a boil then reduce the heat so it bubbles gently. Cook, stirring occasionally, until the vegetables are tender, 10 to 15 minutes. Add a little more stock or water if the mixture gets too dry.

3 Return the chicken to the pan and add the peas, coconut milk, and yogurt. Adjust the heat so the mixture begins to bubble and cook, stirring, until everything is heated through and the sauce thickens, 2 or 3 minutes. Taste and adjust the seasoning; fish out the whole chiles, if you used them. Garnish with the cilantro and scallion greens and serve.

SLOWER CURRY When you add the stock and firm vegetables in Step 2, add the peas, coconut milk, and yogurt, and return the chicken to the pan. Bring to a boil then adjust the heat so that it bubbles gently. Partially cover the pan and cook until the vegetables are very tender but not yet falling apart, about 1 hour. Turn the heat to high for a few minutes to thicken the liquid even more, if you like.

SLOWEST CURRY In this version the vegetables will almost entirely melt into the sauce. Put all of the ingredients in a slow-cooker, stir to combine a bit, and cook on low heat until the chicken and vegetables are very tender, about 6 hours.

NUTRITIONAL INFO *(made with chicken stock, cauliflower, and peas, and served over ¾ cup long-grain brown rice):*
Calories: 496 • Cholesterol: 71mg • Fat: 19g • Saturated Fat: 7g • Protein: 30g • Carbohydrates: 54g • Sodium: 923mg • Fiber: 9g • Trans Fat: 0g • Sugars: 9g

CRISP VEGETABLE AND CHICKEN CUTLETS

MAKES: 4 SERVINGS   TIME: 45 MINUTES

Oven-fried, breadcrumb-topped chicken is way better than the usual fast-food fare, and here you gain crunchy vegetable cutlets in the bargain. Large vegetables with lots of surface area work best: I love celeriac, but winter squash, sweet potatoes, rutabaga, eggplant, or portobello mushroom caps are all wonderful.

6 tablespoons olive oil

¼ cup Dijon mustard

1 teaspoon salt, plus more to taste

Black pepper to taste

2 large or 4 small boneless, skinless chicken breasts (about 1 pound)

1½ pounds celery root, peeled and cut into ¼-inch-thick slices

1½ cups breadcrumbs, preferably whole grain and homemade

Chopped fresh parsley, for garnish

2 lemons, cut into wedges, for serving

1   Heat the oven to 400°F. Divide 2 tablespoons of the oil between two rimmed baking sheets. Combine 2 more tablespoons of oil with the mustard in a small bowl with the salt and lots of black pepper.

2   Put the celery root slices on one of the prepared pans; turn them over a couple times and rub them on both sides until they're coated all over with the oil.

3   If the chicken cutlets are large, cut them so you have four pieces. Put them in the other prepared pan, turn them over a couple times, and rub them on both sides until they're coated all over with the oil. Spread them as flat as you can, pounding them a bit with your fist if you need to. Brush the tops of the celery root and the chicken with the mustard mixture. Sprinkle the breadcrumbs over the celery root and chicken, and lightly press the crumbs down. Drizzle everything with the remaining 2 tablespoons oil, and transfer both pans to the oven.

4   Bake, undisturbed, until both the chicken and celery root are cooked through, 10 to 15 minutes. (You'll be able to pierce the celery root with a fork. Nick the chicken with a knife; it should cut easily and be just

slightly pink inside. If the chicken is thick, it may take a few additional minutes to cook through. If that's the case, remove the celery root from the oven while the chicken finishes cooking.) Garnish with the parsley and serve with lemon wedges.

NUTRITIONAL INFO:
Calories: 579 • Cholesterol: 73mg • Fat: 29g • Saturated Fat: 4g • Protein: 33g • Carbohydrates: 48g • Sodium: 1261mg • Fiber: 6g • Trans Fat: 0g • Sugars: 6g

SUBSTITUTIONS
Instead of the mustard mixture in Step 1, use a different flavoring mixture to help the breadcrumbs stick. Figure 2 to 4 tablespoons total, depending on your taste.

Tomato paste
Chopped fresh herbs
Crumbled dried
  herbs
Pesto
Soy or teriyaki
  sauce

Hoisin
Peanut butter or
  tahini (thinned
  with a little water)
Miso (thinned with a
  little water)

Worcestershire
  sauce
Barbecue sauce
Salsa

HOMEMADE BREADCRUMBS
Everything about homemade breadcrumbs is better: Not only do you choose the bread, you control the texture of the crumbs; coarser are best. Start with whole-grain bread, then cut or break it into 1-inch chunks. If it isn't already on the dry side, let it sit out for several hours or put it in a 200° oven until it's no longer spongy and is just lightly toasted, 20 to 30 minutes. Pulse the dried bread in a food processor or blender, working in batches if necessary, until the crumbs are as coarse or fine as you like. Store in an airtight container at room temperature for several days or in the freezer for months.

STICKS AND STONES

MAKES: 4 SERVINGS   TIME: 1 HOUR, LARGELY UNATTENDED

Instead of a whole bird with a few vegetables scattered around it, roast a few drumsticks with a load of vegetables: both chicken and vegetables become crisp and glazed in their own flavorful juices, and the cooking time is shorter than for a whole bird. If drumsticks aren't your thing, you can substitute chicken thighs or bone-in breast halves.

2 tablespoons olive oil

4 chicken drumsticks (about 1½ pounds)

2 pounds small new or fingerling potatoes, scrubbed but left whole

8 carrots (about ½ pound), cut into 2-inch lengths

8 celery stalks (about ½ pound), cut into 2-inch lengths

A few sprigs of thyme or a branch of rosemary

1 teaspoon salt, plus more to taste

Black pepper to taste

¼ cup chopped fresh parsley or basil, for garnish

Lemon wedges, for serving

1 Heat the oven to 400°F. Drizzle the bottom of a large, shallow roasting pan or a rimmed baking sheet with half of the oil. Add the chicken, vegetables, thyme or rosemary, half the salt, and some pepper, and toss; arrange the chicken skin side up. Roast, undisturbed, until everything is sizzling and starting to turn golden, 20 to 25 minutes.

2 Sprinkle with the remaining ½ teaspoon salt and more pepper, and drizzle with the rest of the remaining tablespoon oil; toss again. Continue to roast, undisturbed, until the vegetables are tender and the chicken is done (its juices will run clear), another 10 to 15 minutes.

3 Remove the thyme or rosemary, sprinkle with the parsley or basil, and serve hot, warm, or at room temperature, with the lemon wedges.

NUTRITIONAL INFO *(with the chicken skin left on)*:
Calories: 567 • Cholesterol: 137mg • Fat: 23g • Saturated Fat: 5g • Protein: 39g • Carbohydrates: 51g • Sodium: 817mg • Fiber: 9g • Trans Fat: 0g • Sugars: 10g

SKILLET SWEET POTATOES WITH SLICED STEAK

MAKES: 4 SERVINGS   TIME: ABOUT 30 MINUTES

The fastest way to cook root vegetables is to grate and stir-fry them. They get tender in a hurry, retaining the slightest crunch while caramelizing in the bargain. The trick is to stir them just enough to prevent burning, but not enough to completely mash them. Sweet potatoes cooked this way are the perfect complement to juicy sliced steak.

3 tablespoons olive oil

2½ pounds sweet potatoes, peeled and grated (about 5 cups)

1 teaspoon salt, plus more to taste

2 tablespoons minced garlic

1 tablespoon chopped fresh sage, marjoram, or oregano (optional)

1 pound beef sirloin, flank, strip, or other steak (about 1 inch thick)

Black pepper to taste

¾ cup red wine or water

1   Heat the oven to 200°F. Put 1 tablespoon of the oil in a large nonstick or cast-iron skillet over medium-high heat. When it's hot, add half of the sweet potatoes, sprinkle with ½ teaspoon salt, and cook, stirring occasionally, until browned in places and almost tender, 3 to 5 minutes. Add 1 tablespoon of the garlic and cook, stirring occasionally, until fragrant, just a minute or two more. Add half of the herb, if you're using it, and stir. Put the potatoes on an ovenproof serving dish and transfer them to the oven to keep warm. Add another tablespoon of oil to the skillet and repeat with the remaining potatoes. Add them to the first batch.

2   Put the remaining tablespoon oil in the skillet and let it get hot. Sprinkle the remaining ½ teaspoon salt and lots of black pepper into the hot fat, and immediately put the steak (or steaks) on top. Cook, undisturbed, until the meat develops a brown crust on the bottom and releases easily, 3 to 5 minutes. Turn and cook until the other side browns a little, too, and the steak is still a little more rare than you like it, no more than a couple more minutes. (The best way to know for sure is to nick the steak with a sharp knife and peek inside.)

3 Transfer the steak to a cutting board, and add the wine to the skillet. Cook, stirring to loosen any browned bits and let the liquid reduce to a little less than ½ cup. Cut the steak across the grain into ½-inch slices and arrange them on top of the potatoes. Pour the pan juices over all and serve.

NUTRITIONAL INFO *(with sirloin steak):*
Calories: 551 • Cholesterol: 67mg • Fat: 17g • Saturated Fat: 4g • Protein: 30g • Carbohydrates: 63g • Sodium: 703mg • Fiber: 10g • Trans Fat: 0g • Sugars: 12g

SUBSTITUTIONS
Instead of the sweet potatoes, try one of these other root vegetables:

Potatoes	Parsnips	Turnips
Winter squash	Rutabaga	Daikon radish
Carrots	Celery root	

BRAISED VEGETABLES AND BEEF

MAKES: 4 SERVINGS   TIME: 1½ HOURS, LARGELY UNATTENDED

The rich, meaty flavor of a good stew doesn't come from using a ton of beef, but from thoroughly browning the amount you do use. This recipe leaves room in the pot for more vegetables, like mushrooms (themselves meaty), carrots and/or parsnips, potatoes, and hearty greens. Simmered slowly with red wine, stock, and herbs, this stew is incredibly satisfying, even without a load of meat.

2 tablespoons olive oil

1 pound boneless beef chuck or round, trimmed and cut into 1-inch cubes

1 teaspoon salt, plus more to taste

Black pepper to taste

1 pound fresh mushrooms (any kind), stemmed if necessary and rough chopped

1 medium onion, chopped

4 carrots or parsnips (or a combination), chopped

1 pound small new or large fingerling potatoes, unpeeled

½ cup red wine

3 cups vegetable stock (see page 241) or water

2 sprigs fresh thyme or rosemary

1 bay leaf

1 pound chopped kale or collards, thick (over-¼-inch) stems discarded

¼ cup chopped fresh parsley, for garnish

1   Put the oil in a large pot over medium-high heat. When it's hot, add the beef, sprinkle with ½ teaspoon salt and lots of pepper, and let it brown until it releases from the pot. Continue to cook, turning the pieces occasionally, until deeply colored on all sides, 5 to 10 minutes total; adjust the heat as necessary and remove the pieces as they are done.

2   Pour off all but 2 tablespoons of the fat and lower the heat to medium. Add the mushrooms, onion, carrots, and potatoes. Add the remaining ½ teaspoon salt and more pepper, and cook, stirring occasionally, until the vegetables begin to brown and stick to the bottom of the pan, 10 to 15 minutes. Add the red wine and cook, stirring to loosen the bits of vegetables, about a minute.

3   Add the stock and return the beef to the pot along with the herb and bay leaf. Bring to a boil, then lower the heat so that the liquid bubbles gently. Cover and cook until the meat is fork-tender and the potatoes are cooked through, 30 to 40 minutes. (You can make the dish to this point up to 3 days ahead; cover and refrigerate, then gently reheat and continue with the recipe.)

4   Stir in the greens and continue cooking until the meat and vegetables are fully tender, 10 to 15 minutes. Add more liquid at any point if the mixture seems dry. Remove the herb sprigs and bay leaf; taste and adjust the seasoning. Garnish with the parsley and serve immediately, or cover and refrigerate for up to 2 days.

BRAISED VEGETABLES AND CHICKEN Substitute 4 bone-in chicken thighs for the beef, browning as above. In Step 3, return the browned chicken to the pot along with the greens, and cook until the chicken is fully cooked (an instant-read thermometer should register 165ºF) and the greens are tender, 15 to 25 minutes.

NUTRITIONAL INFO:
Calories: 464 • Cholesterol: 73mg • Fat: 14g • Saturated Fat: 3g • Protein: 34g • Carbohydrates: 50g • Sodium: 1137mg • Fiber: 10g • Trans Fat: 0g • Sugars: 10g

MEATBALLS, THE NEW WAY

MAKES: 4 SERVINGS   TIME: ABOUT 1 HOUR

Combining grains with vegetables and meat makes for a better meat-ball, moister and more complex in texture and flavor. The combination here is bulgur and spinach, but any soaked or cooked grains (brown rice or steel-cut oats are also nice) work well, as do mashed beans (use about 1½ cups).

There are just as many ways to eat these meatballs as there are to cook them: Put a few on a tossed green salad (page 231), stuff into a pita with sliced cucumbers and tomatoes, or add them to the tomato sauce on page 239 and simmer for a few minutes, then serve with pasta or on toast.

¼ cup medium-grind bulgur

1 cup boiling water

1 pound ground beef, pork, or lamb

1 cup chopped cooked spinach (thawed frozen is fine), squeezed as dry as possible

1 tablespoon minced garlic

1 teaspoon salt, plus more to taste

Black pepper to taste

3 tablespoons olive oil

1 Combine the bulgur and boiling water in a small bowl; cover and soak until fully tender, 15 to 20 minutes. Drain in a strainer, then press out as much of the water as possible. Combine the bulgur, beef, spinach, garlic, and salt and sprinkle with pepper. Shape into 16 meatballs, handling them no more than is necessary.

2 Put the oil in a large skillet over medium heat. When it's hot, add some of the meatballs; work in batches if necessary to avoid overcrowding. Cook, turning once or twice and adjusting the heat as necessary, until they're firm and browned all over, 5 to 10 minutes. As they finish, transfer them to paper towels to drain and repeat with the remaining meatballs as necessary. Serve hot or at room temperature.

NUTRITIONAL INFO *(4 meatballs, made with 80% lean ground beef)*:
Calories: 439 • Cholesterol: 81mg • Fat: 34g • Saturated Fat: 10g • Protein: 23g • Carbohydrates: 10g • Sodium: 609mg • Fiber: 3g • Trans Fat: 1g • Sugars: 0g

SUCCOTASH, GREENS, AND SAUSAGE

MAKES: 4 SERVINGS   TIME: 30 MINUTES

Spike succotash with sausages and a few more vegetables, and you have an easy one-pan meal. Frozen corn is fine here and lets you cook this year-round, though of course fresh corn is even better: Strip the husks from six or eight cobs and carefully cut all the way around with a sharp knife (slicing downward, away from you) to remove the kernels and save as much of their milk as you can. A little apple cider vinegar adds a bright burst of flavor, but you can just as easily use fresh lime or lemon juice. Or, serve the sausages and vegetables alongside thick tomato slices.

> 1½ tablespoons olive oil
>
> 2 sweet or hot Italian sausages (or other fresh sausages, about 6 ounces each), split in half lengthwise
>
> 1½ cups frozen lima or fava beans
>
> 8 scallions, white and green parts separated and chopped
>
> 2 red bell peppers, chopped
>
> 1 tablespoon minced garlic
>
> 2 cups corn kernels (don't bother to thaw if they're frozen)
>
> 1 teaspoon salt, plus more to taste
>
> Black pepper to taste
>
> 4 cups arugula or spinach
>
> 1 tablespoon apple cider vinegar, or more as needed

1 Put ½ tablespoon of the olive oil in a large skillet over medium heat. When it's hot, add the sausage halves and cook, turning as necessary, until browned on both sides and cooked through, 5 to 10 minutes. Remove the sausages from the pan and pour off all but 1 tablespoon of the fat. Meanwhile, put the lima beans in a colander and run them under cold water for a minute or two; set them aside to drain.

2 Raise the heat to medium-high, and add the remaining tablespoon of olive oil to the pan along with the white parts of the scallions, the peppers, and garlic. Cook, stirring occasionally, until the vegetables begin to soften, 2 or 3 minutes. Add the lima beans and the corn, and sprinkle with the salt and some pepper. Cook, stirring occasionally, until the mixture is hot, 3 to 5 minutes.

3   Add the arugula and vinegar and cook, stirring constantly, until the greens soften a little, just a minute or two. Stir in the green parts of the scallions and return the sausages to the pan. Taste and adjust the seasoning, and serve.

SUCCOTASH AND CHICKEN Substitute 4 large boneless chicken thighs for the sausage. Proceed with the recipe.

NUTRITIONAL INFO *(with 3 ounces pork sausage):*
Calories: 524 • Cholesterol: 65mg • Fat: 34g • Saturated Fat: 11g • Protein: 21g • Carbohydrates: 37g • Sodium: 1292mg • Fiber: 7g • Trans Fat: 0g • Sugars: 9g

CABBAGE, SAUERKRAUT, AND PORK CHOPS

MAKES: 4 SERVINGS   TIME: ABOUT 45 MINUTES

Braising sauerkraut along with fresh cabbage takes the edge off of the bracing condiment, and the combination is both powerful and sweet. Here, pork chops are browned to develop their flavor, then simmered along with the cabbage and sauerkraut. The bone helps flavor the broth, and the sliced meat adds texture to the vegetables. This dish is wonderful with bone-in chicken thighs or smoked pork chops.

2 tablespoons olive oil

4 small center-cut bone-in pork chops (about 6 ounces each)

1 large onion, halved and sliced

1 tablespoon minced garlic

1 tablespoon paprika

1 pound green cabbage, cored and shredded

1 pound sauerkraut, preferably fresh or bagged, drained

1½ cups vegetable stock (see page 241), beer, or water

½ teaspoon salt, plus more to taste

Black pepper to taste

1   Put the oil in a large, deep skillet over medium-high heat. A minute later, add the pork chops and cook, turning and adjusting the heat as necessary, until browned on both sides and just cooked through, 5 to 10 minutes total. Remove the pork from the pan.

2   Add the onion and garlic to the pan and cook, stirring, until softened, 3 to 5 minutes. Add the paprika and cook, stirring, until fragrant, about a minute.

3   Add the cabbage, sauerkraut, and stock. Add the salt and sprinkle with pepper and stir. Bring to a boil, then lower the heat so the liquid bubbles gently and cover. Cook, stirring occasionally, until the cabbage is tender but not mushy and the sauerkraut loses some sharpness, 20 to 30 minutes. Nestle the chops in the cabbage mixture and cook just long enough to heat through, 1 or 2 minutes. Taste and adjust the seasoning, and serve with the cooking liquid.

NUTRITIONAL INFO *(with vegetable stock):*
Calories: 490 • Cholesterol: 124mg • Fat: 26g • Saturated Fat: 5g • Protein: 40g •
Carbohydrates: 26g • Sodium: 1129mg • Fiber: 10g • Trans Fat: 0g • Sugars: 9g

11

Building Block Recipes

The recipes in the preceding chapters will help you eat well for months, but those in this chapter will help you eat well forever. These are the core dishes that will change your life, the basics of cooking in a style that takes you away from the SAD and into the world of plant-based eating. They'll show you how easy it is to make VB6 routine and delicious, to make your diet enjoyable, sustainable, infinitely varied, and easy. Once you get the hang of cooking this way—and you quickly will—you'll want to explore and improvise more on your own.

As I've said from the beginning, VB6 is about eating real food, simply prepared. If you already know how to cook, it'll move along faster. But even if you're inexperienced or reluctant, you'll have long-term success by cultivating these three habits:

1. **Prepare and cook food in bulk.** Grouping kitchen tasks makes use of every minute you spend in the kitchen and gives you lots of prepared food that's ready to eat, or to quickly assemble into delicious meals. The key is always to cook with the next meal, and the ones after that, in mind. Whenever you're in the kitchen, waiting for something to cook, ask yourself, "What else could I be doing?" The answer is almost always "plenty": Make a batch of vinaigrette (page 232): boil vegetables for tomorrow's lunch or dinner (page 233);

simmer a pot of beans or grains (pages 236 and 235); trim and rinse a head of lettuce for salad (page 231); or even start a loaf of bread (page 243). This chapter is designed to help get you started thinking of big-picture food preparation and storage. It's easy to be efficient and get in the habit of double-cooking. You'll be rewarded with dinner and something delicious to pack for lunch in the morning.

2. **"Repurpose" leftovers.** Once you have components like salad fixings and cooked vegetables, grains, or beans, your options for snacking and mealtimes expand exponentially. Here's what I mean: Extra tomato sauce can be used as a base for soups or stews; cooked beans can be added to salads or mashed into dip; leftover rice and vegetables make for a lightning-fast stir-fry. Now you're cooking real food more often than not.

3. **Vary the seasonings.** Plainly cooked staples—like the grains, beans, vegetables, and other dishes here—are blank canvases, ready for flavoring with herbs, spices, aromatic vegetables, oils, vinegars, you name it. Keep your pantry and spice cabinet filled with condiments and seasonings (see pages 129 to 135 for some details), and keep some fresh herbs in the fridge, and nothing has to taste the same way twice.

FRUIT COMPOTE

MAKES: 4 SERVINGS   TIME: ABOUT 45 MINUTES

This is among the best ways I know to use fruit that's nearly overripe. And (especially if you skip the sugar), you can enjoy compote freely after meals, for breakfast or snacks, or as part of lunch or dinner.

Almost any fruit will work, alone or in combination: apples, pears, peaches, nectarines, plums, cherries, berries, mangos, pineapple, even citrus. Begin by cooking the firmest fruit, adding in softer ones as the first begin to turn tender, so that the whole thing doesn't turn into mush.

For added flavor, squeeze in a pinch of citrus zest or juice or sprinkle in some chopped basil, mint, or even rosemary toward the end. And compote isn't necessarily sweet (think of chutney): try adding minced garlic, ginger, and chiles; dried spices like curry powder and ground cloves; or even a tiny splash of wine, soy sauce, vinegar, or hot sauce.

> 2 pounds fresh fruit
>
> ½ teaspoon salt
>
> ¼ cup sugar, preferably turbinado (optional)

1. Trim, peel, pit, and seed the fruit as necessary. Cut it into 1- or 2-inch chunks or slices. Combine the fruit and ½ cup water in a saucepan or skillet over medium heat; add the salt and the sugar, if you're using it. When you hear the mixture start to bubble, lower the heat so it barely simmers.

2. Cook, stirring occasionally and adding a splash of water if the mixture gets too dry, until the fruit is tender and the color darkens, 15 to 30 minutes, depending on the fruit. Serve warm or cold, or let the mixture cool completely and store in a covered jar in the refrigerator for up to a week.

PUREED FRUIT Once the fruit is tender, let it cool for a few minutes, then transfer it to a blender or food processor; puree until it reaches the texture you like.

NUTRITIONAL INFO *(for a combination of mangoes, oranges, plums, and pineapple, with sugar)*:
Calories: 175 • Cholesterol: 0mg • Fat: 0g • Saturated Fat: 0g • Protein: 2g • Carbohydrates: 44g • Sodium: 244mg • Fiber: 4g • Trans Fat: 0g • Sugars: 39g

DAILY SALAD BOWL

MAKES: ABOUT 8 3-CUP SERVINGS   TIME: 30 MINUTES

You may think salad must be made at the last minute, but once they're prepped, ready to go, and properly stored, the components last for days in the fridge. Rinse, trim, and chop vegetables that don't discolor or wilt, like celery, carrots, peppers, onions, cucumbers, radishes, and so on, and keep them in a bowl of water. Rinse, tear, dry, and store lettuce in a salad spinner, or in a plastic bag or airtight container lined with a towel. Do this, and keep a jar of your own dressing (page 232) stashed in the fridge, and a fresh salad is never more than a minute away—perfect as a side or with additions that make it a meal.

To vary the ingredients with the season, substitute root vegetables (turnips, rutabagas, or beets) for the cucumbers; celery root for the celery; daikon or jícama for the radishes; and apples, pears, or citrus for the tomato. Instead of lettuce, try ribbons of cabbage (any kind) or raw kale or collards. (You're shooting for about 24 total cups.)

> 8 celery stalks, chopped
>
> 8 carrots, chopped
>
> 1 red onion, chopped
>
> 2 cucumbers, peeled, seeded, and chopped
>
> 2 red or green bell peppers, chopped
>
> 2 bunches radishes, sliced
>
> 2 large heads romaine, torn into bite-size pieces
>
> 2 pints ripe cherry or grape tomatoes, rinsed only
>
> Your Own Salad Dressing (page 232)

1   Prepare the vegetables and lettuce, or prepare them in advance and store them as described in the headnote and ingredient list.

2   Combine as many ingredients as you like, and drizzle about 3 table-spoons of dressing per serving over all. Toss and serve immediately.

NUTRITIONAL INFO *(3 tablespoons):*
Calories: 237 • Cholesterol: 0mg • Fat: 15g • Saturated Fat: 2g • Protein: 5g • Carbohydrates: 24g • Sodium: 309mg • Fiber: 8g • Trans Fat: 0g • Sugars: 13g

YOUR OWN SALAD DRESSING

MAKES: 8 SERVINGS   TIME: 10 MINUTES

Of all the things you can make rather than buy, salad dressing—vinaigrette—is among the easiest, most satisfying, and best. The store-bought stuff often contains scary chemicals and unnecessary sweeteners, and for what you're getting, is outrageously expensive. You can make fresh salad dressing with real ingredients in no more than a couple of minutes, and when you're done you can either use the dressing right away or keep it in the fridge for a week or so.

And dressings are easy to vary: Use sunflower or grapeseed oil for lighter flavor; use any vinegar you like, or try lemon juice; substitute tomato paste for mustard. Instead of water you can add something with more punch, like unsweetened apple juice, vegetable stock, or a bit of soy sauce. And the herb can become a handful of mixed chopped fresh herbs, or curry or chili powder. For spice, try a tiny bit of minced garlic, chiles, or ginger.

> ½ cup olive oil
>
> ½ cup balsamic or any wine vinegar
>
> ¼ cup Dijon mustard
>
> 1 teaspoon dried thyme or tarragon (optional)
>
> ½ teaspoon salt, plus more to taste
>
> Black pepper to taste

Put the oil, vinegar, mustard, and herb, if you're using it, in a small jar with a tight-fitting lid; add ¼ cup water, the salt, and some pepper. Shake vigorously until well combined. Refrigerate for up to a week.

NUTRITIONAL INFO *(3 tablespoons)*:
Calories: 138 • Cholesterol: 0mg • Fat: 14g • Saturated Fat: 2g • Protein: 0g • Carbohydrates: 3g • Sodium: 213mg • Fiber: 0g • Trans Fat: 0g • Sugars: 2g

DAILY COOKED VEGETABLES

MAKES: 8 SERVINGS   TIME: 10 TO 30 MINUTES, DEPENDING ON VEGETABLE

Whether you want a platter of cooked vegetables for a big dinner or a batch to eat throughout the week, this recipe gets the job done for just about any vegetable (the exceptions are eggplant and peppers).

This recipe is essentially a series of guidelines that you can modify to your taste. Some people like their veggies a bit on the crunchy side (which makes them excellent additions to salads or stir-fries), while others like them tender or even downright overcooked (soft vegetables are tremendously useful for purees, sauces, soups, and spreads). If you're planning on storing them for later, but you don't know what you want to do with them yet, err on the less-cooked side. (You can always cook them more.)

I suggest boiling just one kind of vegetable at a time; the timing is much easier than with combinations in the same pot. "Shocking" just-cooked vegetables captures their color and doneness at any stage you like. Here's how: Fill a clean sink or large bowl with ice water. As soon as the vegetables are crisp-tender and vibrantly colored, drain them and plunge them into the ice water; drain again, and wrap tightly to refrigerate or freeze for another time.

One last tip: If you want to eat the thick stems (sometimes called "ribs") of greens like chard, bok choy, kale, collards, and broccoli, separate them from the leaves (or florets, in the case of broccoli), chop them roughly, and begin cooking them 2 or 3 minutes before you start the leaves (or florets)—this way everything will become tender at about the same time.

You can refrigerate cooked vegetables in a covered container for a few days or freeze them for up to a month. Reheat in a microwave, or toss in some oil in a skillet for a couple of minutes.

    2 teaspoons salt, plus more to taste

    About 3 pounds virtually any vegetable

    2 tablespoons lemon juice, plus more to taste

    2 tablespoons olive oil

    Black pepper to taste

    Chopped fresh herbs or ground seasonings (optional)

1 Bring a large pot of water to a boil and add 1½ teaspoons salt. Trim, peel, stem, and seed the vegetables as needed, then cut into big chunks or slices if necessary. When the water boils, put the vegetables in the pot and cook uncovered.

2 Check tender greens after less than a minute; root vegetables will take 10 minutes or more. Everything else is somewhere in between. Every so often while the vegetables are cooking, pluck a piece out with tongs and test it. (With experience, you won't need to do this so often.) Remember that the vegetables will continue to cook a little as they cool.

3 When the vegetables are just a little bit more firm than you ultimately want them, transfer them to a colander to drain. (This is the stage at which you'd shock them if you like; see headnote.) To serve, drizzle with the lemon juice and oil, sprinkle with the remaining ½ teaspoon salt (or more) and some pepper; add more herbs or seasonings you like.

MICROWAVE-COOKED VEGETABLES You'll need to cook the amount of vegetables discussed above in two batches. Put the vegetables on a plate or in a shallow bowl along with a few drops of water; don't drown them. Cover loosely with a paper towel, a vented microwave cooking lid, or a heavy plate. Set the timer for 5 minutes on high, but don't walk away: Timing will depend on your oven's power. Every minute or two, stop the machine and—careful of the steam—poke the vegetables with a thin-bladed knife to check for doneness. When the vegetables are cooked as you like them, proceed as above, serving as you wish, or cooling and storing for later.

COOKED VEGETABLE SALAD Drizzle any cooked vegetables with the dressing on page 232 (or a squeeze of lemon). Serve cold or at room temperature.

NUTRITIONAL INFO *(asparagus):*
Calories: 68 • Cholesterol: 0mg • Fat: 4g • Saturated Fat: 1g • Protein: 4g •
Carbohydrates: 7g • Sodium: 488mg • Fiber: 4g • Trans Fat: 0g • Sugars: 3g

BIG-BATCH RICE AND GRAINS

MAKES: ABOUT 8 1-CUP SERVINGS   TIME: 10 MINUTES TO MORE THAN 1 HOUR

Grains store and reheat so well, there's no reason to cook a small batch. And this formula (I can barely call it a recipe) is all you'll ever need.

The method is forgiving: If you add too little or too much water to the pot, the worst that can happen is that you'll have to add a little more as the grains cook, or drain off the excess when they're done.

Choose from brown rice, bulgur, quinoa, barley, steel-cut oats, millet, cracked wheat, hominy, wheat berries, farro, or wild rice—they'll all cook fine this way, though the timing will be different.

Once they're in the fridge, you'll use them as-is in salads or soups, or reheat them in single or multiple servings. Warm them in the microwave on medium, or in a covered pot on the stovetop with a few drops of water over low heat, or toss in a bit of oil to reheat. You can freeze them, too, for up to a few months; thaw in the fridge or microwave.

3 cups almost any rice or whole grain (about 1¼ pounds)

2 teaspoons salt, plus more to taste

1   Rinse the rice or grains in a strainer and put them in a large pot with the salt. Add enough water to cover by about 1 inch, no more. Bring to a boil, then adjust the heat so the mixture bubbles gently.

2   Cover and cook, undisturbed, until the grains are tender and almost all of the water is absorbed. This will take 5 to 10 minutes for bulgur, 15 to 20 minutes for steel-cut oats, 20 to 25 minutes for quinoa and farro, at least 30 minutes for long-grain brown rice, and 1 hour or more for some specialty rices and sturdy grains like wheat berries or hominy. Add boiling water as needed to prevent sticking and burning.

3   Every now and then, taste; they're done when tender but still a little chewy. If the water is all absorbed (watch for the little holes on the surface), cover the pot and remove it from the heat. If some water still remains but the grains are done, drain them in a strainer, return to the pot, cover, and remove from the heat. They'll stay warm for about 20 minutes. To serve, fluff the grains with a fork. Serve as is or add flavorings (alone or in combination) from the list on page 237.

NUTRITIONAL INFO *(for long-grain brown rice):*
Calories: 257 • Cholesterol: 0mg • Fat: 2g • Saturated Fat: 0g • Protein: 6g • Carbohydrates: 54g • Sodium: 489mg • Fiber: 2g • Trans Fat: 0g • Sugars: 1g

BIG-BATCH BEANS

MAKES: ABOUT 8 ¾-CUP SERVINGS   TIME: 30 MINUTES TO 2 HOURS, DEPENDING ON
THE BEAN AND SOAKING OPTION

Keeping beans handy is one of the best things you can do for your diet, and cooking them yourself is no more difficult than boiling water. (Try it once, and you'll see that they're vastly superior to canned; but also see the sidebar on page 238.) Not only are they full of fiber, protein, and other nutrients, no two kinds are quite the same, making them endlessly versatile. Use them in salads or stir-fries, puree them into dips or sandwich spreads, use them (and their cooking liquid) for soup, or just flavor with any of the ideas in the sidebar on the opposite page.

> 1 pound dried beans, like chickpeas (see the variation for
> lentils and split peas)
>
> 2 teaspoons salt
>
> 1 teaspoon black pepper

1   Rinse the beans under running water, picking through them for stones or debris. Soak them if you have time (see the sidebar). Put in a large pot with enough cold water to cover by about 3 inches. Bring the water to a boil, then reduce the heat so the water barely bubbles. Cover the pot tightly and let the beans cook, undisturbed, for 45 minutes.

2   Try a bean. If it's at all tender, add the salt and pepper. Make sure the beans are still covered by about 1 inch of water; add a little more if necessary. If the beans are still hard, don't add the seasonings yet and make sure they're covered by about 2 inches water.

3   Return the liquid to a gentle bubble and cover. Check for doneness every 10 to 15 minutes and add more water if necessary, enough to keep the beans barely submerged. Small beans will take as little as 15 minutes more; older or large beans can take up to an hour or more. If you haven't added salt and pepper yet, add them when the beans are just turning tender. Stop cooking when the beans are as firm or creamy as you like them. (I like beans more cooked than many people, but it's a matter of taste.) Taste and adjust the seasoning.

4   Now you have a few options. Drain (reserving the liquid separately) to use them as an ingredient in salads or other dishes where they need to be dry, or finish all or some of them with one of the ingredients from the list on the facing page. Then store them: To refrigerate, keep the beans and their cooking liquid in an airtight container; you can always

drain off the liquid as needed, but it's good to keep around if you end up making soup. To freeze, divide the beans into individual or meal-size portions among airtight containers, just covered with cooking liquid. To thaw frozen beans, put them in the refrigerator overnight, in a pot over low heat, or in the microwave. (Beans will keep in the fridge for up to a week and in the freezer for months.)

BIG-BATCH LENTILS OR SPLIT PEAS OR BEANS Follow the directions in the main recipe, but start checking the beans or peas after about 15 minutes. Split peas and beans will break down quickly and inevitably become soupy. (But if you want lentils intact for salads or stir-fries, watch them like a hawk, and drain them the instant they get tender, but before they break open.) Drain, reserving the cooking liquid if you like, and run under cold water to stop their cooking.

BIG-BATCH BEANS IN A SLOW-COOKER Follow the directions in the main recipe, using a slow-cooker set on high. Don't bother to start checking the beans for at least 3 hours, and after that only check them every 30 minutes or so. (You can cook lentils and split beans or peas in a slow-cooker but what you'll get is pretty much soup.)

NUTRITIONAL INFO *(for ¾ cup plain chickpeas):*
Calories: 206 • Cholesterol: 0mg • Fat: 3g • Saturated Fat: 0g • Protein: 11g •
Carbohydrates: 34g • Sodium: 498mg • Fiber: 10g • Trans Fat: 0g • Sugars: 6g

WAYS TO FLAVOR COOKED GRAINS OR BEANS
You probably don't want to flavor the whole pot of grains or beans the same way. It's better—and more interesting—to season the servings to taste as you go.

Chopped fresh tomatoes	Any vinaigrette	Spice blend, like curry or chili
Leftover cooked vegetables, like greens or peppers	Soy sauce	powder
	Olive oil	Minced fresh chile,
	Miso, thinned with a little hot water or cooking liquid	ginger, or garlic
Chopped fresh herbs or crumbled dried herbs		Hot sauce
	Sesame oil	Balsamic or any wine vinegar

HOW TO BUY AND PREPARE BEANS

Dried You can find lots of different kinds in the supermarket, but if you'd like to try heirloom and specialty varieties, check out the bulk offerings in gourmet or natural food stores, or shop online.

I almost never soak beans; in way less than the time it takes you to soak them, you can cook them. But if you think of it, and are leaving the house or going to sleep, you can shorten the cooking time a bit by soaking: Put them in a big pot (or bowl) with enough cold water to cover them by a few inches, and let them sit for up to 12 hours. They'll absorb some liquid, soften and plump a bit, and take a little less time to cook. But if you haven't thought far enough ahead to soak the beans, don't worry about it; just start cooking them as described in the recipe or variations. They'll take a little longer to soften, but require no more attention.

Canned Even though I cook a pot of beans almost every week, I try to keep a couple cans in the pantry; they're fine in a pinch. If you know you won't cook beans from scratch, buy big cans and lots of 'em. You won't find the variety that you'll get with dried, but there's still a good selection, especially in natural food stores. Look for cans that say "BPA Free," which means the lining isn't coated in a type of plastic that might be toxic. And since canned beans are packed in a thick, often quite salty liquid, drain and rinse them well.

Frozen A few kinds of beans—like lima, fava, and black-eyed peas—are available frozen; these cook much faster than their dried counterparts and tend to stay intact longer. Boil them in plenty of salted water, or cook them in a covered container in the microwave. But since the cooking time is so variable, you've got to check them for tenderness frequently.

Fresh If you shop at farmers' markets or specialty stores (or if you garden!), you'll run across fresh beans, in or out of the pod or shell. Fresh peas and fava beans are most common but sometimes you'll see chickpeas, edamame, black-eyed peas, or cranberry beans. These are a treasure, so grab 'em. Cook them like frozen beans, or see the Edamame recipe on page 190.

TOMATO SAUCE WITH LOTS OF VEGGIES

MAKES: 8 1¼-CUP SERVINGS   TIME: ABOUT 90 MINUTES

I love to load this sauce with chopped vegetables, which turns it into something both hearty and healthy, but if you're after a simple marinara, just leave them out. Make sure to explore different fresh and dried herbs, ground spices (tomato sauce with curry served over vegetables or brown rice is a winner), or a splash of red or white wine. For more options—including making your own salsa—see the variations below.

¼ cup olive oil

2 onions, chopped

1 pound mushrooms, chopped

4 carrots, chopped

2 red or green bell peppers, chopped

2 tablespoons minced garlic

1½ teaspoons salt, plus more to taste

Black pepper, or crushed red pepper, to taste

2 28-ounce cans diced tomatoes, with their juice

1 cup chopped fresh basil or ½ cup chopped fresh parsley (optional)

1   Put the oil in a large pot over medium heat. When it's hot add the onions, mushrooms, carrots, bell peppers, garlic, and ½ teaspoon salt, and sprinkle with pepper. Cook, stirring occasionally, until the vegetables are soft and all of their liquid has evaporated, 25 to 30 minutes.

2   Add the tomatoes and the remaining teaspoon salt and adjust the heat so the mixture bubbles steadily. Cook, stirring occasionally, until the tomatoes break down, the vegetables become very soft, and the mixture thickens, 20 to 30 minutes. If the mixture looks too thick, stir in a splash of water.

3   Stir in the basil or parsley, if you're using it; taste and adjust the seasoning and serve. (Or store, tightly covered, in the refrigerator for up to several days, or the freezer for up to several months.)

COOKED SALSA Omit the mushrooms and carrots. Substitute red or white onions for the yellow onions, poblano chiles or minced jalapeños for the bell peppers, and cilantro for the basil. Cook until the tomatoes break down and the heat from the chiles has infused the salsa, 10 to 15 minutes, or longer if you have time. Squeeze in a little lime juice before serving.

MARINARA SAUCE Omit the mushrooms, carrots, and bell peppers. Cook the onion and garlic just to soften, 3 to 5 minutes, then proceed with the recipe.

MEATY TOMATO SAUCE Reduce the olive oil to 2 tablespoons. Start Step 1 by browning 1 pound ground beef, pork, turkey, lamb, or chopped or bulk sausage in the olive oil. Once it loses its pink color add the vegetables (you can stick with just onion and garlic if you like, or include the mushrooms, carrots, and peppers as well), and proceed with the recipe.

NUTRITIONAL INFO *(1¼-cup serving):*
Calories: 152 • Cholesterol: 0mg • Fat: 8g • Saturated Fat: 1g • Protein: 5g • Carbohydrates: 18g • Sodium: 674mg • Fiber: 5g • Trans Fat: 0g • Sugars: 10g

FAST AND FLAVORFUL VEGETABLE STOCK

MAKES: MORE THAN 2 QUARTS   TIME: ABOUT 45 MINUTES

Nowhere is the gap between homemade and store-bought greater than with vegetable stock. The kind you buy in the store tastes so much like water that if I don't have time to make my own—well, I just use water. (Which is fine, in many cases.)

Fortunately, this recipe is both quick and easy, since the mushrooms, tomato paste, and soy sauce (all ingredients that have lots of *umami*, or "savoryness") flavor simmering water faster than meat bones do. But even if you'll just simmer some carrots, celery, and onions in water for 20 minutes, you'll have something infinitely better than what you'd find at the store. If you have a big enough pot, double the recipe and freeze whatever is left. It's most convenient to divide the stock into small serving sizes (or even freeze it in an ice cube tray) so you don't have to thaw out more that you need, although you can always refreeze what you thaw and don't use.

2 medium or 1 large onion, quartered

4 carrots, cut into chunks

2 celery stalks, roughly chopped

1 pound button mushrooms, trimmed but left whole

4 (or more) whole garlic cloves, unpeeled, crushed

1 bunch fresh parsley, stems and leaves

4 sprigs fresh thyme, or a big pinch of dried

1 teaspoon whole black peppercorns

4 bay leaves

¼ cup tomato paste

¼ cup soy sauce

½ teaspoon salt, plus more to taste

Black pepper to taste

1   Combine everything in a stockpot with 3 quarts of water. Bring to a boil and adjust the heat so the mixture bubbles steadily but gently. Cook until the vegetables are tender, about 30 minutes. (If you are in a hurry, you can stop cooking after 20 minutes; if you have a little extra time, let it simmer for an hour, go for it; the flavor will deepen and improve.)

2 Strain the stock, using a spoon to press on the vegetables to extract as much liquid as possible, then taste and add more salt and pepper, if you like. Use right away or cool before storing. (It will keep in the fridge for a week or in the freezer for a few months.)

SLOWER (BUT EVEN MORE FLAVORFUL) VEGETABLE STOCK Roast the onions, carrots, celery, mushrooms, and garlic in a 450°F oven, stirring occasionally, until brown, 30 to 45 minutes. Transfer the roasted vegetables to the stockpot and proceed with the recipe, simmering for 30 minutes or longer.

NUTRITIONAL INFO *(estimated, for 1 cup)*:
Calories: 15 • Cholesterol: 0mg • Fat: 0g • Saturated Fat: 0g • Protein: 0g • Carbohydrates: 3g • Sodium: 640mg • Fiber: 0g • Trans Fat: 0g • Sugars: 2g

D.I.Y. FLATBREAD

MAKES: 8 SERVINGS   TIME: AT LEAST 1 HOUR

Made as a flatbread, this do-it-yourself whole wheat creation falls somewhere on the spectrum between a cracker and a focaccia, with a satisfyingly crunchy crust and some of the airiness that you get from a yeasted loaf bread. But there are many ways to use the dough; see the variations, all of which have a wonderful nutty flavor.

There are different techniques for flavoring: You can add ingredients to the dough with everything else in the food processor; try chopped fresh or crumbled dried herbs, ground spices, minced garlic, ginger, chiles, olives, or dried tomatoes, or even chopped nuts. Or, treat the flatbread like pizza and scatter ingredients on top once the dough is in the pan. This can be as simple as a light drizzle of olive oil or a sprinkle of garlic and herbs, or be an assortment of chopped raw or cooked vegetables, olives, capers, roasted red peppers, or caramelized onions.

In other words, if you can put it on a pizza, you can put it on this flatbread; just make sure to use a light hand with the topping; if you weigh the dough down too much, it won't puff up as it should.

> 3 cups whole wheat flour, plus more for dusting
>
> 1 teaspoon instant yeast
>
> 1 teaspoon salt
>
> 1 cup warm water, plus more as needed
>
> 2 teaspoons olive oil

1   Combine the flour, yeast, and salt in a food processor. Turn the machine on and add the water and 1 teaspoon of the oil through the feed tube. Process until the dough becomes a barely sticky, easy-to-handle ball, about 30 seconds. If it's too dry, add more water a tablespoon at a time, and process for another 10 seconds. If it's too wet (unlikely), add more flour 1 tablespoon at a time. Turn the dough out onto a lightly floured surface, knead it a few times into a ball, and cover with a clean towel until it almost doubles in size, anywhere from 30 minutes up to 2 hours, depending on the room's temperature.

2   Heat the oven to 500°F. Line a baking sheet with parchment paper, and grease the paper with the remaining teaspoon of oil. Roll out the

dough until it's about ⅛ inch thick (the shape doesn't really matter). Carefully transfer the paper and dough to the baking sheet.

3   Bake, reversing the baking sheet once, until the bread is golden and crisp, and has puffed up slightly, 10 to 12 minutes. Cut the bread into 8 pieces, or tear it at the table. Serve hot, warm, or at room temperature. (Whatever you don't eat in a day or two, wrap in foil and store in the freezer. To reheat later, put the still-wrapped frozen bread in a 300°F oven until it thaws and warms, 20 to 30 minutes.)

D.I.Y. SANDWICH BREAD This will be denser and smaller than commercial loaves, but you can slice it thin, and it provides a great base for all sorts of fillings: Grease a 9 x 5-inch loaf pan with 1 teaspoon of olive oil. When the dough has risen, flatten it into a rectangle, then fold the long sides into the middle and pinch them together at the seam. Put the dough in the pan, seam side down, and tuck the short ends underneath so it fits in the pan. Press the dough firmly into the prepared pan. Cover with a towel and let rest until it puffs up again, 30 to 60 minutes. Heat the oven to 350°F. Bake until the top is crusty and the inside is cooked through (the internal temperature should be about 210°F), about 45 minutes. Let cool completely on a wire rack before slicing.

D.I.Y. BREADSTICKS Heat the oven to 400°F. Once the dough has risen and been rolled as described in steps 1 and 2, slice the rectangle into equal pieces about as wide as you want your breadsticks to be. Roll out each piece on a work surface with your hands so that they are the same thickness throughout, as long or short as you want. Put them back on the parchment paper and transfer to the oven. Bake, turning (or rolling) a few times, until they are golden on the outside and cooked through in the middle, 8 to 10 minutes for ¼ inch thick, 10 to 12 minutes for ½ inch, and 12 to 14 minutes for 1 inch. Serve hot, warm, or at room temperature.

D.I.Y. RUSTIC CRUSTY BREAD Heat the oven to 450°F. Put a 2- to 3-quart cast-iron, enamel, ceramic, or Pyrex pot in the oven while it heats. When the oven is hot, carefully remove the pot from the oven and put the round of dough in the pot. Cover the pot and return to the oven. Bake for 20 minutes, then remove the lid and bake until the loaf is beautifully browned, another 15 to 20 minutes. If at any point the bread smells like it's burning, lower the heat. Remove the bread from the pot and let cool completely on a wire rack before slicing.

D.I.Y. FOCACCIA After the dough has risen in Step 1, heat the oven to 500°F and smear a large baking sheet with 1 tablespoon olive oil. Press the dough into the pan, leaving it ¼ to ½ inch thick; dimple the top with your fingertips and sprinkle with salt, pepper, a tablespoon of chopped fresh rosemary, and another tablespoon of olive oil. Cover with a towel and let the dough sit until it puffs nicely, 30 to 60 minutes, depending on the heat of the room. Bake until golden all over and springy to the touch, 15 to 20 minutes. Let cool in the pan before cutting into squares or breaking into pieces.

NUTRITIONAL INFO *(for 1 piece):*
Calories: 165 • Cholesterol: 0mg • Fat: 2g • Saturated Fat: 0g • Protein: 6g • Carbohydrates: 33g • Sodium: 244mg • Fiber: 5g • Trans Fat: 0g • Sugars: 0g

Source Notes

In researching the science of nutrition for this book, I consulted hundreds of studies, journals, online sources, books, and databases, and personally interviewed many renowned experts: scientists, doctors, researchers, on-the-ground field workers, and so on. To save space, we've combined footnotes and a bibliography into a sort of hybrid I hope is more useful. Sources that have directly or indirectly informed the conclusions and observations in my book are listed by first appearance, by chapter. In cases where I had access to a full study that isn't available for free to the general public, a link is provided to the abstract online.

INTRODUCTION

Lipitor website. www.lipitor.com/.

"Statins: Are These Cholesterol-Lowering Drugs Right for You?" www.mayo clinic.com/health/statins/CL00010.

Moyer, Melinda. "It's Not Dementia, It's Your Heart Medication: Cholesterol Drugs and Memory." *Scientific American*, October 19, 2010. www.scientific american.com/article.cfm?id=its-not-dementia-its-your-heart-medication.

Hession, M., Rolland, C., Kulkarni, U., Wise, A., Broom, J. "Systematic Review of Randomized Controlled Trials of Low-Carbohydrate vs. Low Fat/Low-Calorie Diets in the Management of Obesity and Its Comorbidities." *Obesity Reviews.* January 2009; 10(1):36-50. www.ncbi.nlm.nih.gov/pubmed/18700873.

Kolata, Gina. "Low Fat Diet Does Not Cut Health Risks, Study Finds." *New York Times.* February 8, 2006. www.nytimes.com/2006/02/08/health/08fat.html ?pagewanted=all&_r=1&.

Manson, J.E., et al. "Low-Fat Dietary Pattern and Risk of Invasive Breast Cancer: The Women's Health Initiative Randomized Controlled Dietary Modification Trial." *JAMA*, 2006 Feb 8;295(6):629–42. www.ncbi.nlm.nih .gov/sites/entrez?db=pubmed&cmd=historysearch&querykey=2.

Beresford, S.A., et al. "Low-Fat Dietary Pattern and Risk of Colorectal Cancer: The Women's Health Initiative Randomized Controlled Dietary Modification

Trial." *JAMA*. February 8, 2006; 295(6):643–54. jama.jamanetwork.com/
  article.aspx?articleid=202340.
Steinfeld, Henning, et al. "Livestock's Long Shadow: Environmental Issues
  and Options." *FAO*, Rome, 2006. ftp://ftp.fao.org/docrep/fao/010/a0701e/
  a0701e.pdf.

1: THE DIET WITH A PHILOSOPHY

Zuckerbrot, Tanya. *The F-factor Diet: Discover the Secret to Permanent Weight
  Loss*. New York: G.P. Putnam's Sons, 2006.
Kraschnewski, J.L., Boan, J., Esposito, J., Sherwood, N.E., Lehman, E.B.,
  Kephart, D.K., Sciamanna, C.N. "Long-Term Weight Loss Maintenance in the
  United States." *International Journal of Obesity* (Lond). November 2010;
  34(11):1644–54.
Anderson, J.W., et al. "Long-Term Weight Loss Maintenance: A Meta-Analysis
  of US Studies." *American Journal of Clinical Nutrition*, 2001;74:579–84. ajcn
  .nutrition.org/content/74/5/579.full.
Kolata, Gina Bari. *Rethinking Thin: The New Science of Weight Loss—and the
  Myths and Realities of Dieting*. New York: Farrar, Straus, and Giroux, 2007.
University of California Agriculture and Natural Resources. "Global Obesity,
  Child Obesity and Food Consumption/Nutrition." ucanr.edu/News/
  Nutrition,_weight_and_health/Fact_Sheet/.
USDA Agriculture FactBook. "Profiling Food Consumption in America. 2001–
  2002." www.usda.gov/factbook/chapter2.htm.
Census Bureau. "Per Capita Consumption of Major Food Commodities: 1980
  to 2009." Table 217. www.census.gov/compendia/statab/2012/tables/
  12s0217.pdf.
Singer, Peter. *In Defense of Animals: The Second Wave*. Malden, MA: Blackwell
  Pub., 2006.
CDC. "Adult Obesity Facts." www.cdc.gov/obesity/data/adult.html.
Bittman, Mark. "Is Alzhimer's Type 3 Diabetes." *New York Times*, September 25,
  2012. opinionator.blogs.nytimes.com/2012/09/25/bittman-is-alzheimers-
  type-3-diabetes/.
Nestle, Marion, and Nesheim, Malden C. *Why Calories Count: From Science to
  Politics*. Berkeley: University of California Press, 2012.
Block, Gladys. "Foods Contributing to Energy Intake in the US: Data from
  NHANES III and NHANES 1999–2000." *Journal of Food Composition and
  Analysis*, 17 (2004):439–47. itsupport.bvsd.org/schools/FairviewHS/fhsstaff/
  faculty/strode/PIB Bio Course Documents/Unit 4 Human Nutrition and
  Biological Molecules/Foods Contributing to Energy Intake in the US Block
  2004.pdf.
Yang, Sarah. "Nearly One-Third of the Calories in the US Diet Come from
  Junk Food." *UC Berkeley News*, June 1, 2004. berkeley.edu/news/media/
  releases/2004/06/01_usdiet.shtmlhttp://berkeley.edu/news/media/
  releases/2004/06/01_usdiet.shtml.

Nation Master. "Food Statistics. Soft Drink Consumption (most recent) by Country." www.nationmaster.com/graph/foo_sof_dri_con-food-soft-drink-consumption.

Pizza Facts. www.thepizzajoint.com/pizzafacts.html.

USDA Economic Research Service. "Daily Intake of Nutrients by Food Source 2005-2008." www.ers.usda.gov/data-products/food-consumption-and-nutrient-intakes.aspx - 26667.

Daniel, C.R., Cross, A.J., Koebnick, C., Sinha, R. "Trends in Meat Consumption in the USA." *Public Health Nutrition,* April 2011; 14(4): 575-583. www.ncbi.nlm.nih.gov/pmc/articles/PMC3045642/.

"How Much Meat Do We Eat, Anyway?" *Center for a Livable Future.* March 21, 2011. www.livablefutureblog.com/2011/03/how-much-meat-do-we-eat-anyway.

Bittman, Mark. "Rethinking the Meat-Guzzler." *New York Times*, January 27, 2008. www.nytimes.com/2008/0½7/weekinreview/27bittman.html?pagewanted=1&_r=2.

Speedy, A.W. "Global Production and Consumption of Animal Source Foods." *Journal of Nutrition,* November 2003; 133(11 Suppl 2):4048S-4053S. jn.nutrition.org/content/133/11/4048S.full.

Nassauer, Sarah. "The Salad Is in the Bag." *Wall Street Journal*, July 27, 2011. online.wsj.com/article/SB10001424053111903999904576469973559258778.html.

Weight-Control Information Network. "Overweight and Obesity Prevalence Estimates, 2008." www.win.niddk.nih.gov/statistics/index.htm - overweight.

NCHS Data Brief. "Prevalence of Obesity in the United States, 2009-2010," January 2012. www.cdc.gov/nchs/data/databriefs/db82.pdf.

CDC. "Obesity at a Glance, 2011." www.cdc.gov/chronicdisease/resources/publications/aag/obesity.htm.

CDC. "Prevalence of Obesity Among Children and Adolescents: United States, Trends 1963-1965 Through 2007-2008." www.cdc.gov/nchs/data/hestat/obesity_child_07_08/obesity_child_07_08.htm.

Lustig, Robert. *Fat Chance: Beating the Odds Against Sugar, Processed Food, Obesity, and Disease.* New York: Hudson Street Press, 2013.

Langreth, R., Stanford, D. "Fatty Foods Addictive as Cocaine in Growing Body of Science." *Bloomberg BusinessWeek*, November 11, 2011. www.businessweek.com/news/2011-11-11/fatty-foods-addictive-as-cocaine-in-growing-body-of-science.html.

Garber, A.K., Lustig, R.H. "Is Fast Food Addictive?" *Curr Drug Abuse Rev.* September 2011; 4(3):146-62. Review. www.ncbi.nlm.nih.gov/pubmed/21999689.

Yale Rudd Center for Food Policy and Obesity. "Fast Food Facts: Evaluating Fast Food Nutrition and Marketing to Youth," November 2010. grist.files.wordpress.com/2010/11/fastfoodfacts_report.pdf.

Brown, David. "Study: 42% Likely to Be Obese by 2030." *USA Today*, May 8, 2012. www.usatoday.com/USCP/PNI/Nation/World/2012-05-08-PNI0508wir-obesity_ST_U.htm.

Steinfeld, Henning, et al. "Livestock's Long Shadow: Environmental Issues and Options." *FAO*, Rome, 2006. ftp://ftp.fao.org/docrep/fao/010/a0701e/a0701e.pdf.

FAO Newsroom. "Livestock a Major Threat to Environment." November 29, 2006. www.fao.org/newsroom/en/news/2006/1000448/index.html.

Natural Resources Defense Council (NRDC). "Saving Antibiotics: What You Need to Know About Antibiotics Abuse on Farms." August 3, 2012. www.nrdc.org/food/saving-antibiotics.asp.

FAO Agriculture and Consumer Protection Department. "Livestock Impacts on the Environment," November 2006. www.fao.org/ag/magazine/0612sp1.htm.

FAO Compassion in World Farming. "Global Warning: Climate Change and Farm Animal Welfare," 2008. www.fao.org/fileadmin/user_upload/animal welfare/GlobalWarningExecutiveSummary1.pdf.

Hill, Holly. "Food Miles: Background and Marketing." *National Sustainable Agriculture Information Service*, 2008. attra.ncat.org/attra-pub/farm_energy/food_miles.html.

Pimentel, David, and Pimentel, Marcia. *Food, Energy, and Society.* Niwot, CO: University of Colorado, 1996.

Humane Society of the United States. "Farm Animal Statistics: Meat Consumption," November 30, 2006. www.humanesociety.org/news/resources/research/stats_meat_consumption.html.

"Vegetarianism in America." *Vegetarian Times.* www.vegetariantimes.com/article/vegetarianism-in-america/.

"A Handful of Companies Controls the Food Industry," Diagram. www.convergencealimentaire.info.

Yale Rudd Center for Food Policy and Obesity. "Fast Food Facts: Evaluating Fast Food Nutrition and Marketing to Youth," November 2010. grist.files.wordpress.com/2010/11/fastfoodfacts_report.pdf.

Welch, G. "Spending in the U.S. on Advertising for Fast Foods, Sodas, and Automobiles: Food for Thought Regarding the Type 2 Diabetes Epidemic." *Diabetes Care,* February 2003; 26(2): 546. care.diabetesjournals.org/content/26/2/546.full.

Gallo, Anthony. "Advertising in the United States." USDA/ERS. www.ers.usda.gov/media/91050/aib750i_1_.pdf.

World Public Health Nutrition Association. "What Drives Global Obesity?" *World Nutrition,* Volume 3, Number 6, June 2012. www.wphna.org/2012_june_wn2_editorial.htm.

"Kids Get Diet of Junk Food Commercials." *CBS News,* March 30, 2010. www.cbsnews.com/2100-204_162-2620036.html.

Brownell, Kelly D., and Battle, Katherine Horgen. *Food Fight: The Inside Story of the Food Industry, America's Obesity Crisis, and What We Can Do About It.* Chicago: Contemporary, 2004.

Federal Trade Commission. "FTC Report Sheds New Light on Food Marketing to Children and Adolescents," July 29, 2008. www.ftc.gov/opa/2008/07/foodmkting.shtm.

Wansink B. *Mindless Eating: Why We Eat More Than We Think.* New York: Bantam, 2010.

Reisner, Rebecca. "The Diet Industry: A Big Fat Lie?" *Bloomberg BusinessWeek*, January 10, 2008. www.businessweek.com/debateroom/archives/2008/01/ the_diet_indust.html.

U.S. Department of Commerce Industry Report. "Food Manufacturing." NAICS, 311. trade.gov/td/ocg/report08_processedfoods.pdf.

Slim Fast nutrition information. www.slim-fast.com.

Nestlé nutrition information for a Kit Kat. www.nestle.ca.

LeanCuisine nutrition facts. www.leancuisine.com.

Davis, William. *Wheat Belly: Lose the Wheat, Lose the Weight, and Find Your Path Back to Health.* Emmaus, PA: Rodale, 2011.

Ebbeling, C.B., Swain, J.F., Feldman, H.A., et al. "Effects of Dietary Composition on Energy Expenditure During Weight-Loss Maintenance." *JAMA.* 2012; 307(24):2627-2634. jama.jamanetwork.com/article.aspx?articleid=1199154.

Spake, A. "The Science of Slimming," *U.S. News & World Report,* June 26, 2003: 34-40. health.usnews.com/usnews/health/articles/030616/16 weight.htm.

The Cabbage Soup Diet. www.cabbage-soup-diet.com.

Atkins Website. www.atkins.com/Home.aspx.

Phone conversation with Ludwig, June 23, 2012.

Polivy, J., Coleman, J., Herman, C.P. "The Effect of Deprivation on Food Cravings and Eating Behavior in Restrained and Unrestrained Eaters." *International Journal of Eating Disorders*, 2005; 38:301-309. www.ncbi.nlm .nih.gov/pubmed/16261600.

Yancy, W.S., et al. "A Low-Carbohydrate, Ketogenic Diet Versus a Low-Fat Diet to Treat Obesity and Hyperlipidemia: A Randomized, Controlled Trial." *Annals of Internal Medicine*, May 18, 2004; 140(10): 769-77. www.ncbi.nlm.nih .gov/pubmed/15148063.

Kong, A., et al. "Self-Monitoring and Eating-Related Behaviors Are Associated with 12-Month Weight Loss in Postmenopausal Overweight-to-Obese Women." *Journal of the Academy of Nutrition and Dietetics*, September 2012; 112(9):1428-35. www.andjrnl.org/article/S2212-2672%2812%2900634-X/ abstract.

Hollis, J.F., et al. Weight Loss Maintenance Trial Research Group. "Weight Loss During the Intensive Intervention Phase of the Weight-Loss Maintenance Trial." *American Journal of Preventive Medicine.* August 2008; 35(2):118-26. www.ncbi.nlm.nih.gov/sites/entrez?db=pubmed&cmd=historysearch& querykey=1.

"Best Diets: Weight Watchers Diet." *U.S. News Health.* health.usnews.com/ best-diet/weight-watchers-diet.

Harvard Health Publications. "Money Talks: Financial Incentives for Health." May 2011. www.health.harvard.edu/newsletters/Harvard_Mens_Health_ Watch/2011/May/money-talks-financial-incentives-for-health.

John, L.K., et al. "Financial Incentives for Extended Weight Loss: A Randomized, Controlled Trial." *Journal of General Internal Medicine*, June 2011;

206(6):621–6. www.ncbi.nlm.nih.gov/sites/entrez?db=pubmed&cmd=history search&querykey=3.

"Study Reveals Staggeringly Successful Weight Loss Strategy for Men." *Globe Newswire*, April 10, 2012. www.globenewswire.com/newsroom/news.html?d=251535.

2: WHY VB6 DOES WORK

CDC. "Adult Obesity Facts." www.cdc.gov/obesity/data/adult.html.

Nestle, Marion, and Nesheim, Malden C. *Why Calories Count: From Science to Politics*. Berkeley: University of California, 2012.

Alcock, J., Franklin, M., and Kuzawa, C.W. "Nutrient Signaling: Evolutionary Origins of the Immune-Modulating Effects of Dietary Fat." *The Quarterly Review of Biology* 87:3 (March 2013). www.jstor.org/stable/10.1086/666828.

Dunn, Ron. "The Hidden Truths about Calories." *Scientific American*, August 27, 2012. blogs.scientificamerican.com/guest-blog/2012/08/27/the-hidden-truths-about-calories/.

Barr, S.B., Wright, J.C. "Postprandial Energy Expenditure in Whole-Food and Processed-Food Meals: Implications for Daily Energy Expenditure." *Food & Nutritional Research*. July 2, 2010; 54. doi: 10.3402/fnr.v54i0.5144. www.ncbi.nlm.nih.gov/pmc/articles/PMC2897733/.

Carmody, R.N., Weintraub, G.S., Wrangham, R.W. "Energetic Consequences of Thermal and Nonthermal Food Processing." *Proceedings of the National Academy of Science*. 2011 Nov 29;108(48):19199-203. www.pnas.org/content/108/48/19199.short.

Bee, Peta. "Don't Count Calories, It'll Just Make You FATTER! Which Foods Really Make Us Fat?" *Daily Mail*, September 10, 2012. www.dailymail.co.uk/health/article-2201280/Calories-dont-count-calories-itll-just-make-fatter-which-foods-really-make-fat.html.

Nestle, Marion, and Nesheim, Malden C. *Why Calories Count: From Science to Politics*. Berkeley: University of California Press, 2012.

Mayo Clinic "Energy density and weight loss: Feel full on fewer calories." www.mayoclinic.com/health/weight-loss/NU00195.

USDA National Nutrient Database for Standard Reference. ndb.nal.usda.gov/.

CDC. "Diet/Nutrition," March 29, 2012. www.cdc.gov/nchs/fastats/diet.htm.

Schleicher, Jerry. "Potato Use: All About America's Favorite Vegetable." *Grit Magazine*, June 2010. www.grit.com/vegetables/potato-use-all-about-americas-favorite-vegetable.aspx.

USDA Economic Research Service. "Potatoes," May 28, 2012. www.ers.usda.gov/topics/crops/vegetables-pulses/potatoes.aspx.

Northern Plains Potato Growers Association (NPPGA). "Potato Fun Facts." www.nppga.org/consumers/funfacts.php.

FatSecret Calories and Nutrition for French Fries. www.fatsecret.com/calories-nutrition/usda/french-fries-(in-vegetable-oil)?portionid=62704&portionamount=42.

Wansink B. *Mindless Eating: Why We Eat More Than We Think.* New York: Bantam, 2010.

Nabisco nutrition facts for Wheat Thins. www.nabiscoworld.com.

Frito-Lay nutrition facts for Doritos Salsa Verde Chips. www.fritolay.com.

Harvard School of Public Health. "The Nutrition Source:Carbohydrates." www.hsph.harvard.edu/nutritionsource/what-should-you-eat/carbohydrates/.

Lustig, Robert. *Fat Chance: Beating the Odds Against Sugar, Processed Food, Obesity, and Disease.* New York: Hudson Street Press, 2013.

CDC. "National Diabetes Fact Sheet," 2011. www.cdc.gov/diabetes/pubs/pdf/ndfs_2011.pdf.

U.S. National Library of Medicine. "Hypoglycemia," June 27, 2012. www.ncbi.nlm.nih.gov/pubmedhealth/PMH0001423/.

Suzuki, K., et al. "The Role of Gut Hormones and the Hypothalamus in Appetite Regulation." *Endocrine Journal,* 2010; 57:359-72. www.ncbi.nlm.nih.gov/pubmed/20424341.

Flier, Jeffrey, et al. "What's in a Name? In Search of Leptin's Physiologic Role." *Journal of Clinical Endocrinology and Metabolism* 83, 1407-13 (1998). jcem.endojournals.org/content/83/5/1407.full.

Lustig, R.H., et al., "Obesity, Leptin Resistance, and the Effects of Insulin Suppression." *International Journal of Obesity* 28, 1344-8 (2004). www.ncbi.nlm.nih.gov/pubmed/15314628.

Kellerer, M., et al., "Insulin Inhibits Leptin Receptor Signaling in HEK293 Cells at the Level of Janus Kinase-2: A Potential Mechanism for Hyperinsulinaemia-Associated Leptin Resistance." *Diabetologia* 44, 1125-32 (2001). www.ncbi.nlm.nih.gov/pubmed/11596667.

Klockener, T., et al., "High-Fat Feeding Promotes Obesity Via Insulin Receptor/PI3K-Dependent Inhibition of SF-1 VMH Neurons." *Nature Neuroscience.* 14, 911-8 (2011). www.ncbi.nlm.nih.gov/pubmed/21642975.

Friedman, J.M., Halaas, J.L. "Leptin and the Regulation of Body Weight in Mammals." *Nature* 395:763-70 (2008). www.nature.com/nature/journal/v395/n6704/full/395763a0.html.

Hill, J.W., et al., "Acute Effects of Leptin Require PI3K Signaling in Hypothalamic Proopiomelanocortin Neurons in Mice." *Journal of Clinical Investigation,* 2008. 118, 1796-805. www.ncbi.nlm.nih.gov/pubmed/18382766.

U.S. National Library of Medicine. "Metabolic Syndrome," June 2, 2012. www.ncbi.nlm.nih.gov/pubmedhealth/PMH0004546/.

Sweet Surprise. "What Is High Fructose Corn Syrup?" www.sweetsurprise.com/what-is-hfcs.

Parker, Hilary. "A Sweet Problem: Princeton Researchers Find that High-Fructose Corn Syrup Prompts Considerably More Weight Gain." *Princeton University*, March 22, 2010. www.princeton.edu/main/news/archive/S26/9½2K07/.

Taubes, Gary. *Why We Get Fat: And What to Do About It.* New York: Anchor, 2011.

Mayo Clinic. "Added Sugar: Don't Get Sabotaged by Sweeteners." www.mayoclinic.com/health/added-sugar/MY00845.

ReduceTriglycerides.com. "Triglycerides-Lowering Diet: What About Fructose?" www.reducetriglycerides.com/reader_triglycerides_high_fructose_fruit.htm.

California Wheat Commission. "A Kernel of Wheat." www.californiawheat.org/industry/diagram-of-wheat-kernel/.

USDA Choose My Plate. "What Foods Are in the Grains Group?" www.choose myplate.gov/food-groups/grains.html.

Harvard School of Public Health. "The Nutrition Source: Fiber." www.hsph.harvard.edu/nutritionsource/what-should-you-eat/fiber/.

Mayo Clinic. "Fiber." www.mayoclinic.com/health/fiber/NU00033/.

USDA Healthy Meals Resource System. "High Fiber Foods List and Tips to Increase." healthymeals.nal.usda.gov/hsmrs/Montana/FiberFoodsList.pdf.

Harvard School of Public Health. "The Nutrition Source: Carbohydrates." www.hsph.harvard.edu/nutritionsource/what-should-you-eat/carbohydrates/.

Foster-Powell, K., Holt, S. H., Brand-Miller, J. C. "International table of glycemic index and glycemic load values: 2002." *American Journal of Clinical Nutrition.* 2002 Jul;76(1): 5-56. ajcn.nutrition.org/content/76/1/5.full.

Glycemic Index Database, The University of Sydney. www.glycemicindex.com/.

Harvard Health Publications. Glycemic Index and Glycemic Load for 100 + Foods. www.health.harvard.edu/newsweek/Glycemic_index_and_glycemic_load_for_100_foods.htm.

South Beach Diet. "South Beach Glycemic Index Food Chart." www.south beach-diet-plan.com/glycemicfoodchart.htm.

"Glycemic Indexes." *The Montignac Method.* www.montignac.com/en/search-for-a-specific-glycemic-index/.

Whole Grains Council website. www.wholegrainscouncil.org.

Liu S, Manson JE, Stampfer MJ, et al. "A Prospective Study of Whole-Grain and Risk of Type 2 Diabetes Mellitus in US Women." *American Journal of Public Health,* 2000; 90:1409–15.

www.ncbi.nlm.nih.gov/pubmed/10983198.

Liu, S., et al. "Whole-Grain Consumption and Risk of Coronary Heart Disease: Results from the Nurses' Health Study." *American Journal of Clinical Nutrition,* September 1999; 70(3): 412-9. ajcn.nutrition.org/content/70/3/412.abstract.

Pereira, M., et al. "Effect of Whole Grains on Insulin Sensitivity in Overweight Hyperinsulinemic Adults." *American Journal of Clinical Nutrition,* 2002; 75:846–55. ajcn.nutrition.org/content/75/5/848.full.pdf.

Newby, P.K., et al;. "Intake of Whole Grains, Refined Grains, and Cereal Fiber Measured with 7-d Diet Records and Associations with Risk Factors for Chronic Disease." *American Journal of Clinical Nutrition,* 2007 86: 6 1745-1753. www.ncbi.nlm.nih.gov/pubmed/18065595?dopt=Abstract.

Liu, S. "Whole-Grain Foods, Dietary Fiber, and Type 2 Diabetes: Searching for a Kernel of Truth." *American Journal of Clinical Nutrition,* 2003 77: 3 527-529. ajcn.nutrition.org/content/77/3/527.full.

Mars nutrition information. www.marshealthyliving.com/whats-inside.

Phone conversation with Ludwig, June 23, 2012.

Kolata, Gina Bari. *Rethinking Thin: The New Science of Weight Loss--and the Myths and Realities of Dieting*. New York: Farrar, Straus, and Giroux, 2007.

Harvard School of Public Health. "The Nutrition Source: Fats." www.hsph. harvard.edu/nutritionsource/what-should-you-eat/fats-full-story/index.html.

Pepino, M.Y., Love-Gregory, L., Klein, S., Abumrad, N.A. "The Fatty Acid Translocase Gene, *CD36*, and Lingual Lipase Influence Oral Sensitivity to Fat in Obese Subjects." *Journal of Lipid Research*, Dec. 31, 2011. www.jlr.org/content/early/2011/12/31/jlr.M021873.abstract

Mattes, R.D. "The Taste of Fat Elevates Postprandial Triacylglycerol." *Physiol Behav*, 2001 Oct; 74(3):343-8. www.ncbi.nlm.nih.gov/pubmed/11714498

Shape Up America. "Everything You Want to Know About Body Fat." www.shapeup.org/bfl/basics1.html.

Yale Medical Group. "Why Fat Cells Are Important." www.yalemedicalgroup .org/stw/Page.asp?PageID=STW001874.

WhereInCityMedical. "Fat Facts." www.whereincity.com/medical/fats/.

"Percent Body Fat Calculator." *The American Council on Exercise*. www.acefitness.org/calculators/bodyfat-calculator.aspx.

Fit Day."Percentage Body Fat & Weight—What's Normal?" www.fitday.com/fitness-articles/fitness/weight-loss/percentage-body-fat-weight---whats-normal.html - b.

"Essential Body Fat Should Account for What Percentage of Body Weight in Women?" *Livestrong*. www.livestrong.com/article/258497-essential-body-fat-should-account-for-what-percentage-of-body-weight-in-women/.

Casiday, R., Frey, R. "Nutrients and Solubility." *Washington University Department of Chemistry*. www.chemistry.wustl.edu/~edudev/LabTutorials/Vitamins/vitamins.html.

Tulane University. "Endocrine System: Types of Hormones." e.hormone.tulane .edu/learning/types-of-hormones.html.

Harvard Health Publications. "Vitamins and Minerals: Understanding Their Role." www.helpguide.org/harvard/vitamins_and_minerals.htm.

Kolata, Gina. "Study Finds That Fat Cells Die and Are Replaced." *New York Times*, May 5, 2008. www.nytimes.com/2008/05/05/health/research/05fat .html?_r=2&.

Park, Madison. "When You're Losing Weight, Where Does The Fat Go?" *CNN Health*, July 22, 2011. www.cnn.com/2011/HEALTH/07/22/fat.weight.loss/index.html.

"Do Fat Cells Last Forever?" *CNN Health*, December 2, 2008. articles.cnn. com/2008-12-02/health/fat.cells_1_fat-cells-fat-children-liposuction?_s=PM:HEALTH.

USDA Agriculture FactBook. "Profiling Food Consumption in America. 2001-2002." www.usda.gov/factbook/chapter2.htm.

Wright, J.D., Wang, C.Y. "Trends in intake of energy and macronutrients in adults from 1999-2000 through 2007-2008." Hyattsville, MD: *National Center for Health Statistics*; November 2010. www.cdc.gov/nchs/data/databriefs/db49.htm.

American Heart Association. "About Cholesterol." www.heart.org/
HEARTORG/Conditions/Cholesterol/AboutCholesterol/About-Cholesterol_
UCM_001220_Article.jsp.

Gilhuly, Kathryn. "Can High Blood Pressure Cause High Cholesterol?"
Livestrong, April 22, 2011. www.livestrong.com/article/425976-can-high-
blood-pressure-cause-high-cholesterol/ - ixzz21qWGHyqD.

Anderson, J., Young, L., Roach, J. "Cholesterol and Fats." *Colorado State
University Extension*, December, 2008. www.ext.colostate.edu/pubs/
foodnut/09319.html.

Prentice, R.L., et al. "The Big Fat Question." *Tufts Journal*, January 6, 2010.
tuftsjournal.tufts.edu/2010/01_1/features/03/.

Harvard School of Public Health. "The Nutrition Source: Ask the Expert
Omega-3 Fatty Acids." www.hsph.harvard.edu/nutritionsource/questions/
omega-3/index.html.

Mensink, R., et al. "Effects of Dietary Fatty Acids and Carbohydrates on
the Ratio of Serum Total to HDL Cholesterol and on Serum Lipids and
Apolipoproteins: A Meta-Analysis of 60 Controlled Trials." *American
Journal of Clinical Nutrition*, 2003; 77:1146-55. www.ncbi.nlm.nih.gov/
pubmed/12716665.

Hu, F., Manson, J., Willett, W. "Types of Dietary Fat and Risk of Coronary Heart
Disease: A Critical Review." *Journal of the American College of Nutrition*, 2001;
20:5-19. www.ncbi.nlm.nih.gov/pubmed/11293467.

Lacroixd E., et al. "Randomized Controlled Study of the Effect of a Butter
Naturally Enriched in Trans Fatty Acids on Blood Lipids in Healthy Women."
American Journal of Clinical Nutrition, February 2012; 95(2):318-25. ajcn
.nutrition.org/content/early/2011/12/28/ajcn.111.023408.abstract.

CDC. "Trans Fats."www.cdc.gov/nutrition/everyone/basics/fat/transfat.html.

Mozaffarian, D., Micha, R., Wallace, S. "Effects on Coronary Heart
Disease of Increasing Polyunsaturated Fat in Place of Saturated Fat:
A Systematic Review and Meta-Analysis of Randomized Controlled
Trials." *PLoS Med*,2010;7:e1000252. www.plosmedicine.org/article/
info%3Adoi%2F10.1371%2Fjournal.pmed.1000252.

Ebbeling, C.B., et al. "Effects of Dietary Composition on Energy Expenditure
During Weight-Loss Maintenance." *JAMA*. 2012;307(24):2627-2634. http://
jama.jamanetwork.com/article.aspx?articleid=1199154.

Riserus, U., Willett ,W.C., Hu, F.B. "Dietary Fats and Prevention of Type 2
Diabetes." *Progress in Lipid Research*, 2009; 48:44-51. www.ncbi.nlm.nih.gov/
pmc/articles/PMC2654180/.

Jakobsen, M.U., et al. "Intake of Carbohydrates Compared with Intake of
Saturated Fatty Acids and Risk of Myocardial Infarction: Importance of the
Glycemic Index." *American Journal of Clinical Nutrition*, 2010; 91:1764-8. www.
ncbi.nlm.nih.gov/pubmed/20375186.

Hu, F.B. "Are Refined Carbohydrates Worse than Saturated Fat?" *American
Journal of Clinical Nutrition*, 2010; 91:1541-2. www.ncbi.nlm.nih.gov/pmc/
articles/PMC2869506/?tool=pubmed.

Hoenig, M.R., Sellke, F.W. "Insulin Resistance is Associated with Increased Cholesterol Synthesis, Decreased Cholesterol Absorption and Enhanced Lipid Response to Statin Therapy." *Atherosclerosis*, July 2010; 211(1):260-5. www.ncbi.nlm.nih.gov/pubmed/20356594.

Hooper, L., et al. "Reduced or Modified Dietary Fat for Preventing Cardiovascular Disease." *Cochrane Database of Systematic Reviews*, 2011: CD002137. www.ncbi.nlm.nih.gov/pubmed/21735388.

Siri-Tarino, P.W., et al. "Saturated Fatty Acids and Risk of Coronary Heart Disease: Modulation by Replacement Nutrients." *Current Atherosclerosis Reports*, 2010; 12:384-90. www.ncbi.nlm.nih.gov/pubmed/20711693.

Harvard School of Public Health. "The Nutrition Source: Protein." www.hsph .harvard.edu/nutritionsource/Printer%20Friendly/Protein.pdf.

Census Bureau. "Per Capita Consumption of Major Food Commodities: 1980 to 2009." Table 217. www.census.gov/compendia/statab/2012/tables/ 12s0217.pdf.

Food and Nutrition Board. "Dietary Reference Intakes for Energy, Carbohydrate, Fiber, Fat, Fatty Acids, Cholesterol, Protein, and Amino Acids (Macronutrients)," 2005. www.nap.edu/openbook.php?isbn=0309085373.

Hicks, J. Morris., and J. Stanfield. Hicks. *Healthy Eating, Healthy World: Unleashing the Power of Plant-Based Nutrition*. Dallas, TX: BenBella, 2011.

Harvard School of Public Health. "The Nutrition Source: Protein." www.hsph .harvard.edu/nutritionsource/questions/protein-questions/index.html #howmuch.

McDougall, John A., and McDougall, Mary A. *The McDougall Plan*. Clinton, NJ: New Win Pub., 1983, page 39.

USDA Choose My Plate. "What Foods Are In the Grains Group?" www.choose myplate.gov/food-groups/grains.html.

Hicks, J. Morris., and J. Stanfield. Hicks. *Healthy Eating, Healthy World: Unleashing the Power of Plant-based Nutrition*. Dallas, TX: BenBella, 2011, page 54.

Ornish, Dean. *Dr. Dean Ornish's Program for Reversing Heart Disease*. New York: Random House, 1990.

Weil, Andrew, M.D. *Natural Health, Natural Medicine*. Boston: Houghton Mifflin, 1998.

Jenkins, D.A., et al. "Effect of Legumes as Part of a Low Glycemic Index Diet on Glycemic Control and Cardiovascular Risk Factors in Type 2 Diabetes Mellitus: A Randomized Controlled Trial." *Archives of Internal Medicine*, 2012. www.ncbi.nlm.nih.gov/pubmed/23089999.

"Lifestyle, Diet and Disease: Early Findings from Adventist Health Study-2." *Loma Linda University School of Public Health*, 2009. Retrieved October 31, 2012. www.llu.edu/public-health/health/lifestyle_disease.page.

Hill, A.J., Blundell, J.E. "Macronutrients and Satiety: The Effects of a High Protein or High Carbohydrate Meal on Subjective Motivation to Eat and Food Preferences." *Nutrition and Behavior*, 3:133–144,1986. openagricola.nal.usda. gov/Record/FNI87001220.

Rolls, Barbara J., and Barnett, Robert A. *Volumetrics Weight-Control Plan: Feel Full on Fewer Calories*. New York: Quill, 2000.

Zuckerbrot, Tanya. *The F-factor Diet: Discover the Secret to Permanent Weight Loss*. New York: G.P. Putnam's Sons, 2006.

Astrup, A., Vrist, E., Quaade, F. "Dietary Fiber Added to Very Low Calorie Diet Reduces Hunger and Alleviates Constipation." *International Journal of Obesity*. (1990) 14:105-112. www.ncbi.nlm.nih.gov/pubmed/2160441.

Burley, V.J., Leeds, A.R., Blundell, J.E. "The Effect of High and Low-Fiber Breakfasts on Hunger, Satiety and Food Intake in a Subsequent Meal." *International Journal of Obesity*. 11 (1987) (suppl. 1): 87-93. www.ncbi.nlm.nih .gov/pubmed/3032830.

Porikos, K., Hagamen, S. "Is Fiber Satiating? Effects of a High Fiber Preload on Subsequent Food Intake of Normal-Weight and Obese Young Men." *Appetite*, 1986 7:153-162. www.ncbi.nlm.nih.gov/pubmed/3017204.

Burton-Freeman, B. "Dietary Fiber and Energy Regulation." *The American Society for Nutritional Sciences. Journal of Nutrition*, February 1, 2000, vol. 130 no. 2 272. http://jn.nutrition.org/content/130/2/272.full.pdf+html.

Flood-Obbagy, J.E., Rolls, B.J. "The Effect of Fruit in Different Forms on Energy Intake and Satiety at a Meal." *Appetite*, 2009. 52:416-422. www.ncbi .nlm.nih.gov/pubmed/19110020.

Bolton, R.P., Heaton, K.W., Burroughs, L.F. "The Role of Dietary Fiber in Satiety, Glucose, and Insulin: Studies with Fruit and Fruit Juice." *American Journal of Clinical Nutrition*, February 1981; 34(2):211-7. www.ncbi.nlm.nih.gov/ pubmed/6259919.

Rolls, B.J., et al. "Volume of Food Consumed Affects Satiety in Men." *American Journal of Clinical Nutrition*, 1998. 67:1170-1177. ajcn.nutrition.org/ content/67/6/1170.full.pdf+html.

Ello-Martin, J.A., et al. "Dietary Energy Density in the Treatment of Obesity: A Year-Long Trial Comparing Two Weight-Loss Diets." *American Journal of Clinical Nutrition*, 2007. 85:1465-1477. ajcn.nutrition.org/content/85/6/1465 .abstract.

Rolls, B.J., Roe, L.S., Meengs, J.S. "Portion Size Can Be Used Strategically to Increase Vegetable Consumption in Adults." *American Journal of Clinical Nutrition*, 2010. 91:913-922. www.ncbi.nlm.nih.gov/pubmed/20147467.

Rolls, B.J., Roe, L.S., Halverson, K.H., Meengs, J.S. "Using a Smaller Plate Did Not Reduce Energy Intake at Meals." *Appetite*, 2007. 49:652-660. www.ncbi.nlm.nih.gov/pubmed/17540474.

Spill, M.K., Birch, L.L., Roe, L.S., Rolls, B.J. "Serving Large Portions of Vegetable Soup at the Start of a Meal Affected Children's Energy and Vegetable Intake." *Appetite*, 2011. 57:213-219. www.ncbi.nlm.nih.gov/ pubmed/21596073.

Flood, J.E, Rolls, B.J. "Soup Preloads In a Variety of Forms Reduce Meal Energy Intake." *Appetite*, 2007 49:626-634. www.ncbi.nlm.nih.gov/pmc/ articles/PMC2128765/.

Knutson, K.L., Van Cauter, E. "Associations Between Sleep Loss and Increased Risk of Obesity and Diabetes." *Annals of the New York Academy of Science*, 2008; 1129:287-304. www.ncbi.nlm.nih.gov/pubmed/18591489.

Rolls, Barbara J., and Barnett, Robert A. *Volumetrics Weight-Control Plan: Feel Full on Fewer Calories*. New York: Quill, 2000.

Snoek, H.M., Huntjens, L., Van Gemert, L.J, De Graaf, C., Weenen, H. "Sensory-Specific Satiety in Obese and Normal-Weight Women." *American Journal of Clinical Nutrition,* October 2004; 80(4):823-31. ajcn.nutrition.org/content/80/4/823.full.

Miller, D.L., et al. "Effects of Dietary Fat, Nutrition Labels, and Repeated Consumption on Sensory-Specific Satiety." *Physiology & Behavior,* 2000; 71:153-158. www.ncbi.nlm.nih.gov/pubmed/11134697.

Bell, E.A., Roe, L.S., Rolls, B.J. "Sensory-Specific Satiety Is Affected More by Volume than by Energy Content of a Liquid Food." *Physiology & Behavior,* April 2003; 78(4-5):593-600. www.ncbi.nlm.nih.gov/pubmed/12782213.

MacRae, Fiona. "Always Have Room for a Dessert? Here's Why: Brain's Pleasure Centers Override Chemicals That Say We Are Full." *Daily Mail,* July 26, 2012. www.dailymail.co.uk/health/article-2179547/Always-room-dessert-Heres-brains-pleasure-centres-override-chemicals-say-full.html.

Wansink, B., Tal, A., Shimizu, M. "First Foods Most: After 18-Hour Fast, People Drawn to Starches First and Vegetables Last." *Archives of Internal Medicine,* 2012; 172(12):961-963. archinte.jamanetwork.com/article.aspx?articleid=1195521.

Redden, Joseph P., and Kelly L. Haws (2013). "Healthy Satiation: The Role of Decreasing Desire in Effective Self-Control," *Journal of Consumer Research,* forthcoming. Article Stable. www.jstor.org/stable/10.1086/667362.

Knutson, K.L., Van Cauter, E. "Associations Between Sleep Loss and Increased Risk of Obesity and Diabetes." *Annals of the New York Academy of Sciences,* 2008; 1129:287-304. www.ncbi.nlm.nih.gov/pubmed/18591489.

Brondel, L., et al. "Acute Partial Sleep Deprivation Increases Food Intake in Healthy Men." *American Journal of Clinical Nutrition,* June 2010; 91(6):1550-9. ajcn.nutrition.org/content/91/6/1550.short.

Donga, E., et al. "A Single Night of Partial Sleep Deprivation Induces Insulin Resistance in Multiple Metabolic Pathways in Healthy Subjects." *Journal of Clinical Endocrinology,* June 2010; 95(6):2963-8. www.ncbi.nlm.nih.gov/pubmed/20371664.

3: THE SIX PRINCIPLES OF VB6

Cascio, Jamais. "The Cheeseburger Footprint." *Open the Future.* openthefuture.com/cheeseburger_CF.html.

"What's in Cheez Whiz—Easy Cheese?" *EduBlog,* January 22, 2009. nutrition.edublogs.org/2009/0½2/whats-in-easy-cheese/.

Kong, A., et al. "Self-Monitoring and Eating-Related Behaviors Are Associated with 12-Month Weight Loss in Postmenopausal Overweight-to-Obese

Women." *Journal of the Academy of Nutrition and Dietetics*, September 2012; 112(9):1428-35. www.andjrnl.org/article/S2212-2672%2812%2900634-X/abstract.

Substance Abuse and Mental Health Services Administration website (SAMHSA) family.samhsa.gov/

Oregon Department of Agriculture. "Eating Out or at Home, Food Is a Bargain for US Consumers." May 23, 2012. cms.oregon.gov/ODA/docs/pdf/news/120523consumption.pdf.

Harvard School of Public Health. "The Nutrition Source: Fats." www.hsph.harvard.edu/nutritionsource/what-should-you-eat/fats-full-story/index.html.

Centers for Disease Control and Prevention. "About BMIs for Adults." www.cdc.gov/healthyweight/assessing/bmi/adult_bmi/index.html.

Harvard School of Public Health. "How to Get to Your Healthy Weight." www.hsph.harvard.edu/nutritionsource/healthy-weight/healthy-weight-full-story/index.html.

Rush University Medical Center. "What Is Healthy Weight?" www.rush.edu/rumc/page-1108048103230.html.

"Diets Don't Work." *Scientific American*, April 5, 2007. www.scientificamerican.com/podcast/episode.cfm?id=BE73BA72-E7F2-99DF-325F60B2E1AB3C7F.

Kanarek, R.B., D'Anci, K.E., Jurdak, N., Mathes, W.F. "Running and Addiction: Precipitated Withdrawal in a Rat Model of Activity-Based Anorexia." *Behavioral Neuroscience,* August 2009; 123(4):905-12. www.ncbi.nlm.nih.gov/pubmed/19634951.

Church, T.S., et al. "Changes in Weight, Waist Circumference and Compensatory Responses with Different Doses of Exercise Among Sedentary, Overweight Postmenopausal Women." *PLoS One*. 2009; 4(2):e4515. www.plosone.org/article/info:doi/10.1371/journal.pone.0004515.

Myers, J. "Cardiology Patient Pages. Exercise and Cardiovascular Health." *Circulation*, January 7, 2003; 107(1):e2-5. circ.ahajournals.org/cgi/content/full/107/1/e2.

Brody, Jane. "Even More Reasons to Get a Move On." *New York Times*, March 1, 2010. www.nytimes.com/2010/03/02/health/02brod.html.

4: EATING VB6

Healthfinder.gov. "Quit Smoking." healthfinder.gov/prevention/printtopic.aspx?topicid=24.

Acknowledgments

The idea of a plant-based diet, a plant-reliant diet, a less-meat, less-junk diet—whatever you want to call it—can take many forms. But in any case, the plant-heavy diet is an idea whose time has come, and VB6 is a simple discipline anyone can manage and therefore, we hope, a valuable aid toward developing a sensible diet.

Happily, I can honestly lay claim to it and, equally happily, I had some of the best inspiration, most capable help, and most wonderful support imaginable.

The inspiration began with Sid Baker, and you've read the story of Sid and me in the introduction. He's been a doctor, a good friend, and a guide to me and many of my loved ones for more than thirty-five years now, and I'm forever and increasingly in his debt. (I love him, actually.)

Kerri Conan, my book-writing partner of nearly ten years, is not exactly "help"; as with Sid, without her, there is no VB6, at least not in book form. But she and I have been living this diet, separated by geography but bound by intent and philosophy and daily contact, for more than six years. And with each passing month we learn more and experience more; it makes more sense to us, and so our commitment grows. We have both worked daily on *VB6* for a long time, and it's as much her book as mine.

Much heavy and graceful lifting was done by Suzanne Lenzer, Laura Anderson, Daniel Meyer, Elena Goldblatt, Meghan Gourley, and Eve Turow. These are talented, smart, lovable people we've come to respect and adore, and all of them have bright futures, filled with Sweetness and Light. Blessings!

Clarkson Potter has been behind *VB6* from the start, and for that we have to thank primarily the great Pam Krauss, with whom I've wanted to work since we were young'uns. We've finally made it happen, and this is the first of many books we'll be doing together. Working with Potter has also reunited me with the world's second greatest publicist (stay with me), Kate Tyler. And it's introduced me to a host of new and wonderful colleagues, including Mark McCauslin, Stephanie Huntwork, Kevin Garcia, Donna Passannate, Anna Mintz, Carly Gorga, and Jessica Freeman-Slade.

I had support in this work from more people than I can count or remember, old friends and colleagues and new. Among those at the *Times* are my (evidently lifelong) editor Trish Hall, Sam Sifton, Hugo Lindgren, George Kalogerakis, Chris Conway, Maureen Muenster, and Jennifer Mascia. Little of this writing would have happened without the help and advice of Andy Rosenthal, Bill Schmidt, Bill Keller, Rick Berke, Laura Chang, and Erica Goode. Outside, I've sought and received wisdom from Ricardo Salvador, Marion Nestle, Michael Pollan, and—again—many others. Their experience, I hope, is evident in these pages, but of course any errors in fact or judgment are mine.

Kerri would like to thank her husband, Sean Santoro (who is enthusiastic and supportive both before and after 6:00), and her gracious New York hosts, Wendy and Kim Marcus.

As I age, life seems to become more rather than less intense, so personal support becomes more important than ever. For this I rely on a number of people: Angela Miller is more friend than agent; John Willoughby is more brother than friend. My children, Kate (the world's greatest publicist) and Emma, are a near-daily source of joy—what a trip! My parents, bless them, continue to pull for me. Finally, there is Kelly, with whom every minute is precious—and there will never be enough of them.

Index

Greens. *See also specific greens*
  and Beans Soup, 164–65
  Braised Vegetables and Beef,
    222–23
  Braised Vegetables and Chicken,
    223
  Creamed, on Toast, 169
  Daily Salad Bowl, 231
  Green Salad with Macerated Fruit
    and Nuts, 158
  Kale Chips Lacinato, 184
  for snacks, 183
  Succotash, and Sausage, 225–26
  Succotash and Chicken, 226
  and Tofu Soup, 165
  washing and storing, 183
Guacamole
  Double Green, 188
  Spiked, 188

H
Heart disease, 16
Herbs, 130–31
High blood pressure, 55
High-density lipoproteins (HDL), 55,
  58, 59
High fructose corn syrup (HFCS),
  42–43
Highly processed foods. *See also* Junk
  food
  addictive nature of, 16
  adverse effect on home cooking,
    19
  candy bar vs. fruit, 50
  convenience of, 19
  cutting consumption of, 75–77, 102
  diet bar vs. candy bar, 20
  effect on cholesterol levels, 58
  environmental impact of, 17–19
  frozen diet lunch vs. VB6 lunch, 21
  hidden sugars in, 43
  high fructose corn syrup in, 42
  limiting, in VB6 diet, 102
  marketing of, 16, 18–22
  profitability of, 35
  in Standard American Diet, 15, 27

store-bought chips vs. homemade
  chips, 37
type of calories in, 32
weight-loss products, 19–22
Wheat Thins vs. wheat berries, 36
Hoecakes
  Corny, 151–52
  Fluffy, 152
  Whole Wheat, with Fruit, 151
Home cooking. *See* Cooking at home
Hunger hormones, 40–42
Hypoglycemia, 40
Hypothalamus, 41

I
Insulin
  glycemic index and, 47–51
  glycemic load and, 49–51
  and hunger hormones, 40–42
  physiological function of, 40–41
  resistance, 40
  secretion of, 39, 42, 47

J
Jam
  Spiced Apple (With or Without
    Toast), 145
  Spiced Tomato, 145
Jerky, Tofu, 189
Junk food
  cutting consumption of, 75–77, 102
  fats in, 54
  in Standard American Diet, 15
  vegan, note about, 185

K
Kale Chips Lacinato, 184
Ketosis, 25

L
Labels. *See* Food labels
Legumes. *See also* Bean(s)
  Big-Batch Lentils or Split Peas or
    Beans, 237
  for flexible pantry, 132
  Lentil Salad, 159

M